A Self-Determined Future with Asperger Syndrome

of related interest

The Complete Guide to Asperger's Syndrome
Tony Attwood
ISBN 978 1 84310 495 7
eISBN 978 1 84642 559 2

An Asperger Dictionary of Everyday Expressions
2nd edition
Ian Stuart-Hamilton
ISBN 978 1 84310 518 3
eISBN 978 1 84642 578 3

Asperger Syndrome – A Love Story
Sarah Hendrickx and Keith Newton
Foreword by Tony Attwood
ISBN 978 1 84310 540 4
eISBN 978 1 84642 662 9

How to Find Work that Works for People with Asperger Syndrome
The Ultimate Guide for Getting People with Asperger Syndrome into the Workplace (and keeping them there!)
Gail Hawkins
ISBN 978 1 84310 151 2

Asperger's Syndrome
A Guide for Parents and Professionals
Tony Attwood
Foreword by Lorna Wing
ISBN 978 1 85302 577 8
eISBN 978 1 84642 697 1

Asperger Syndrome and Bullying
Strategies and Solutions
Nick Dubin
Foreword by Michael John Carley
ISBN 978 1 84310 846 7
eISBN 978 1 84642 635 3

A Self-Determined Future with Asperger Syndrome

Solution Focused Approaches

E. Veronica Bliss and Genevieve Edmonds

Foreword by Bill O'Connell

Jessica Kingsley *Publishers*
London and Philadelphia

First published in 2008
by Jessica Kingsley Publishers
116 Pentonville Road
London N1 9JB, UK
and
400 Market Street, Suite 400
Philadelphia, PA 19106, USA

www.jkp.com

Library of Congress Cataloging in Publication Data

Bliss, E. Veronica.
A self-determined future with Asperger syndrome : solution focused approaches / E. Veronica Bliss and Genevieve Edmonds.
p. cm.
Includes bibliographical references and index.
ISBN-13: 978-1-84985-550-1 (alk. paper) 1. Asperger's syndrome--Patients--Rehabilation. 2. Solution-focused therapy. I. Edmonds, Genevieve. II. Title.
RC553.A88B59 2007
616.85'883206--dc22

2007021767

British Library Cataloguing in Publication Data

A CIP catalogue record for this book is available from the British Library

ISBN 978 1 84985 550 1
eISBN 978 1 84642 685 8

Printed and bound in the United States

For both our mums and dads who always told us we could. Except when we asked 'Could we have ponies?', in which case they said we most definitely could not.

Contents

Acknowledgements

There is an autistic world out there to whom we are indebted for providing such rich, entertaining and sensible material from which we can consolidate old ideas as well as grow new ones. With specific regard to this book, those individuals who have worked so hard and well with us within therapy, teaching situations and social settings are very close to our hearts. Marina Whiteside has been a tower of fun and strength when both of us were simply using words randomly in an effort to describe the indescribable. Marina's son TJ was also a source of much inspiration. For example, it was he who taught us, through his own bitter experience never, *ever* to laugh when you've got hand cuffs on. Fiona Barnett has helped both of us keep the horses warm, dry and fed when there was simply too much work for us to do alone. Neil Shepherd kindly put his mental health at further risk by reading and commenting on drafts which were seriously repetitive, and he found ways of keeping humour alive in the midst of despair. And finally Dominic Bray, who seemed to know all along that we would successfully reach the end of this project. You are all heroes and we thank you profusely.

Both of us also want to thank the animals who form our consulting and therapy team. Dyson the cat marked important passages with paw prints and kept the computer mouse under strict control. Henry the bouncing Border Collie helped with background research that involved quite a surprising amount of ball catching. Grace and Dan, the Irish Draught horses listened to all the highs and lows while remaining ever solution focused and philosophical.

Last, but not least, Vicky better thank Phil, her husband. She gives the old man a lot of grief, but he's the one who, despite working an insane number of hours at his own business, makes sure the home fires are maintained. (Though he never does take out the rubbish and she kind of wishes he would.)

Special Note

We have done our best to provide well written, accurate information within this book. The opinions and views belong to us and we are entirely responsible for the content. We do not produce this book as something which, if followed, will automatically lead to success, and as such we do not accept liability for any difficulties which may arise as the result of an interpretation made by a reader.

Foreword

Solution focused practitioners help people find sustainable solutions. They do this by promoting service users' awareness of their strengths, competencies and personal qualities. Instead of focusing on why people have problems, they invest more time in exploring how people overcome difficulties and manage their lives.

This book graphically describes how the solution focused approach can build respectful and empowering relationships. It is unusual for two reasons – it is a collaborative enterprise between a former service user and her therapist, and secondly the narrative is punctuated with self-deprecating humour.

The book raises many uncomfortable questions for professionals. Vicky and Genevieve challenge many of the assumptions which professionals make about people with AS. They question the degree of power professionals exercise over service users. They are passionately committed to making the voices of service users heard and acknowledged and their unique insights and behavioural strategies understood and accepted.

Being on the cutting edge is rarely a comfortable experience. Vicky, the therapist, finds that the views about service users which some other professionals hold are very different from her own judgements and perceptions. Genevieve bravely shares her mixed experience of the helping professions in order to facilitate change and understanding.

The solution focused model emphasizes working collaboratively within the client's frame of reference. This is particularly relevant in relationships with people with AS who have their own unique ways of seeing and experiencing the world. This book witnesses how clients can experience a sense of liberation when they meet a therapist who validates their world-view and values their insights and strategies.

Being solution focused is more than just using techniques. It embraces a philosophy and a set of values which underpin the therapist's thinking and the kind of relationship she creates with a service user.

The book describes how innovative and life-affirming the approach can be in the hands of a skilled practitioner. As a collaboration between a therapist and a service-user, this book serves as a valuable model of how powerful and illuminating a mutually respectful relationship between a therapist and a service user can be.

I hope the ideas in this book will stimulate readers to respect and validate diversity; focus more on solutions than problems and notice what's working in someone's life rather than what is not working. The practical resources in Chapter Seven will be useful to hard-pressed practitioners and will hopefully be an encouragement to them to develop their skills and knowledge by seeking out opportunities for further training.

Bill O'Connell
Director of Training
Focus on Solutions Ltd

Chapter One

Introduction

What's this book all about, then?

Consider the following: I hate supermarket shopping. Supermarkets provide a mind-ripping distraction for absolutely *all* of one's senses.

First, supermarkets have obscenely bright lighting which often flickers and which *always* causes the bright colours of packaging and advertising to jump and dance before my eyes. The jagged colours then reflect up again from the shiny floors for a second visual assault. I have to squint in an attempt to decrease the amount of light and colour coming into my eyes.

Second, the noise level is positively incapacitating. There are people sounds: the rumble, rumble, blurb, blurb sounds of everyday conversations punctuated by piercing screaming and other high-pitched noises of children, followed by the piercing screaming and lower-pitched but louder noises of their parents. On top of the people sounds, there is a layer of beeping checkout sounds, a layer of swishing and rattling packets topped off with a layer of various clicks, squeaks and buzzes. All of these mainly chaotic and unpredictable sounds are wrapped in jangling music punctuated with sudden, brain-jarring tannoy announcements. I want to cover my ears, but I settle for involuntary jerks of my head in an attempt to clear a path for coherent thought.

Third, there are smells that mix and mingle throughout the building: coffee, baking bread, raw meat, fish, body odours, toilets, photo chemicals, shampoo, perfumed soaps, air fresheners and candle smells. Often these smells merge into tastes in my mouth, which makes me want to scrape my tongue on my teeth for a distraction. Some of the nicer smells take my attention away from what I am trying to do, and if I am not careful, I wander towards the smell and disorient myself.

Fourth, there is a very high degree of demented activity within a supermarket. There are constantly moving people, and the smaller the person, the faster and more unpredictably they move. There are children running, arms reaching, trolleys rolling, paper flapping, things falling, people bumping and items being shifted from shelf to trolley to conveyor belt to bags and back into the trolley again. Honestly, I could weep. It is like uncontrolled dodge 'ems in my mind. I over- or underestimate my distance from people, trolleys, shelves or displays, with the end result of bouncing and banging recklessly down each aisle, like Tigger on amphetamines, flinging assorted apologies and 'oopses' as I go. Happily, the trail of destruction behind me is always worse in my imagination than it is in reality – so far.

Amongst all this, while squinting, jerking my head, scraping my tongue on my teeth and bouncing from one thing to another, I am meant to focus on the reason I came to the supermarket. Somehow, my written list is supposed to grab and hold my attention amid this assault on my senses. I am supposed to be able to switch squinting eyes from my written list to the items on shelves while avoiding any 'odd' behaviour that might, though calming to me, upset, offend or downright frighten other shoppers.

Just picture it! There I am, clutching my list in an ever dampening fist, narrowing my eyes, jerking, twitching, stopping and starting erratically, saying 'cereal', 'sorry', 'sorry', 'oops' to myself between tongue scraping and jerking commando-like among the ebb and flow of people, trolleys and products in the aisles. I take quick glances up every few seconds to orient myself, looking for clues, and I allow myself a little puff of pride and shameless relief as I find the cereal aisle. Ha! Bust my buttons and blow me down – I have arrived without incident. After a little mental 'high five-ing' I have to do some new mental gymnastics in order to make a choice between twenty-five different brands of cereal, at least ten of which are in blue-coloured boxes like the one I am looking for. After making a choice and taking a deep, cleansing breath, I Tigger-bounce off to do the same thing again in the bread aisle.

All this I have learned to do, and then (cue scary organ music) someone recognizes me. Not only do they recognize me, they want, for reasons I simply cannot understand, to *talk* to me. They apparently want conversation in the middle of chaos! Why? Why, for heaven's sake, *why*, in the middle of this war on my senses, in the middle of this magnificent effort of concentration would anyone want to *talk*?! Unless, of course, they need to tell me my hair is on fire or something and then OK...I'll allow for that. But most conversations in supermarkets are, it seems to me, a pointless distraction which is pretty high up the list of 'Things I don't need' when I am already battered by thousands of distractions.

'Hello Vicky! I didn't expect to see you in this neck of the woods.' I jerk to a stop. I am caught. Caught like a rabbit in headlights and I cannot form a word. I can only stare and do a few frantic teeth-on-tongue scrapes.

'Are you going to the meeting?' Meeting? I think the word in synch with my rapid blinking trying to access a useful reference point in my head. My squinting eyes go back and forth, I jerk my head to empty it of sounds, I steady myself on the nearest shelf, then I zero in again on the woman who has interrupted me. Finally I say the word out loud: 'Meeting?' I suddenly wonder (rather oddly under the circumstances) if I am blinking a lot more than is considered normal, and I guess that I am.

'Yes' this big jolly woman says. 'The meeting on the twenty-first.' Again I mentally repeat the phrase but it connects with nothing, as my mind is ripped away by some happy family noises in dairy products that have suddenly grabbed my attention. I say again 'Meeting…?' Squint, jerk, scrape.

'This month!' she exclaims. She seems bizarrely keen about this meeting.

'The meeting on the twenty-first of this month?' I parrot after her. I wonder silently what month of the year it is, and notice that there are no clues of this between cereals and dairy products. I hear a little mental 'snap' and my mind becomes angry. I can almost see my patience dripping into a puddle on the floor. For heaven's sake! Is it necessary to play twenty questions with me? What does this woman want to know? And furthermore, now that I think about it, who is she? Where have I seen her before? Fortunately the safety switch my mum and I installed years ago is still working and my brain and my mouth are disconnected. I am unable to say the things my mind is thinking, so I continue staring at her. Squint, blink, jerk, twitch.

'You said you would come! You said you would be there!' she says, showing no obvious sign of being irritated with my lack of response or my physical quirks. Sadly, there is also no sign of her noticing the tortuous twisting, turning and fatigue of my poor, tired brain cells, though I continue the squinting, jerking and funny mouth movements and I know I am starting to sweat.

'November! It's November' I say, suddenly brightening because my mind has solved one of the many tests being set. 'There is a meeting on the twenty-first of November…in Manchester…yes. Yes, I will be going. Will you?' I ask not because I am even a teeny tiny bit interested in the answer, but because I know asking a question will get me off the hook and buy me some time to calm my over-excited innards. Thankfully, she answers with a paragraph of words, none of which I can process but all of which give me time to try to smooth the spikes out of my brain and construct an escape. The pressure is off me. I repeat a few things she says, I smile, I nod (this is what normal people do) and then my foot shoots out in a tentative effort to make a break for it. I think I finish with a sentence that she possibly finds peculiar because she gives me a look as if she is worried I may be having a stroke. I suddenly wonder why I am not. All of this two-minute exchange takes a heroic effort from my brain, and a stroke about now would make perfect sense. I shuffle off and wander through the brightly coloured aisles, wondering what I am doing in this hell. And I never do buy the bread.

Err...so what's this book about, then?

This book is about noticing how people with minds like mine (though my 'autism' is as yet undiagnosed) manage to negotiate supermarkets, along with other seemingly impossible aspects of everyday living. If you are reading this because you want to support someone who has an Autistic Spectrum Disorder (ASD)[1] or, more specifically to this book, Asperger Syndrome (AS),[2] then this book is about noticing, naming and using the strategies people with AS already employ to get through their days. It is about developing a respectful working partnership with someone whose mind may work in unexpected ways, sometimes different and sometimes similar to yours. It is about working hard to listen to what a person with AS says, and believing that, for them, what they say is true, makes sense, and is the best way they have of cooperating with you at that moment in time, even if you don't understand or agree with it. It is about using language with a common meaning to construct a future which is important to the person with AS, and it is about using that common language to decide how both of you will know when you are doing the right things to move in the direction of the person's preferred future. This book is about you learning to function within an occasionally foreign culture which you need to respect and leave intact, unless you are specifically requested to do otherwise.

1 Autistic Spectrum Disorder as used in this book refers to people who fulfil the diagnostic criteria of: a) difficulty processing non-verbal language, and thus difficulty with communication and social cues; b) difficulty processing sensory information, and thus proneness to self-stimulating behaviour or all-encompassing interests in a few topics; c) difficulty in knowing what is in another person's mind, and thus vulnerability to people who have less than honest intentions, and a tendency toward factual information rather than pretend. ASD is a term used to encompass the full spectrum of autism, from people who need quite a lot of daily support to people who appear to need very little support.

2 Asperger Syndrome, as used in this book, refers to people who appear to need very little daily life support, and have the impairments of ASD.

If you are reading this book as a person with AS, this book is about doing the above things with people who do not have AS. They need your respect, help and understanding too.

This book is *not* about supermarkets, which is probably lucky for all of us. It is also *not* about assuming that people with AS mean the same things as non-autistic people do when they use a word or phrase, or when they set a goal for themselves. It is *not* about assuming that you, as a carer or something similar, know what is best for them, or that you know what they need to do in order to feel better. This book is *not* about assuming there is something 'wrong' with people who have AS (even those who seem rarely happy or impossibly anxious), that needs to be 'dug out' and 'fixed'. It is *not* about assuming that the professional or the non-autistic way is best, or that people with AS need to be 'normalized' in order to fit in to their communities. This book is not even about assuming that people with AS need help from other people, or that they wish to change how they are or what they do. If something isn't broken, this book is about how *not* to fix it.

Again, if you have AS and are reading this book, replace the term 'AS' with 'neurotypical' (NT) and the book will retain its meaning all the same.

The reason supermarkets were even mentioned in the first place is because they represent a big collection of things many people with AS find difficult about ordinary life. Brightness, noises, smells, distractions, movements and feelings that are integral parts of getting through the day can cause a person with AS to become exhausted with the effort of holding it together and getting their needs met. A shopping experience described from an AS point of view, such as the one at the beginning of this chapter, illustrates how different a common experience can be from that of someone who does not have AS. One description is not wrong, it is only different. The person without AS does not have to set out to 'change' the person with AS in order to make shopping a delightful experience for them. In the main, the person without AS can help most by not assuming that everyone does or should experience shopping in the same way as they do, and by being flexible with their thinking in order to understand the possible differences in perceptions.

Another way the person without AS can help is by noticing the heroic efforts being made by the person with AS in order to survive the world *and* get things done. The easiest way to do this is by asking the person with AS how they manage an assault on their senses, such as the supermarket, and still come out with groceries. By asking how they continue to make themselves return to do even more shopping on a regular basis. By asking them to tell you how they experience shopping, then believing what they say. This book is about helping people without AS to do these very things.

Vicky

I am, by way of belated introduction, Veronica Bliss. My brothers, I am told, started calling me Vicky when I was very young and that nickname has stayed with me, causing untold problems with banks, doctors, solicitors and other important institutions, not to mention problems with regular folk knowing me as either Veronica or Vicky, but not as both. (Thank you, brothers of mine. I needed a few more complications in my life.) I am writing from my perspective as someone who clearly hates shopping, and perhaps more importantly, from my experience as a psychologist working with people who have ASD and, more specifically in this book, AS. The people with whom I work often have things labelled depression, anxiety, obsessions, compulsions, or various and sundry other labels alongside or instead of AS.

I used to work with these issues (notice the language there: I used to work with 'issues' rather than people) from a problem focused point of view, assuming that I knew many things about the best way to 'fix' the problems of someone with ASD. I assumed they wanted to be more 'normal' and set about developing programmes of relaxation and learning social skills that would make them fit in with the crowd a bit better. I had an unconscious mindset that if I did not show the client how to behave more normally, they would not change their current problematic behaviour. If they did not change their problematic behaviour, they would not conform to, or fit in with, their own community, and thus they would never be happy. In short, I believed they needed my expert help, and that it was my job to know how to 'fix' them. My toolkit for fixing a person with AS largely involved trying to teach them to recognize and name their emotions (using terms from neurotypical language such as 'happy, sad, guilty', etc.) plus teaching them to recognize the interplay between their thoughts, their behaviours and their feelings, in a pretty standard cognitive behavioural therapy (CBT) format.

Since 2001, however, I have been using a solution focused (de Shazer *et al.* 1986) way of working, which uses a different set of assumptions. I now assume that change is inevitable, that problems do not happen all the time, that people are basically capable individuals who know what works for them, and that people have the basis for positive change already occurring in their lives. My job as a therapist is to listen very closely for evidence of existing strengths, coping skills and important points of view that have helped the person get to where they are today. My job is also to facilitate a joint discussion where we think how to use the person's existing skills to achieve what they want to achieve, and to help the person identify some benchmarks so that we will both know if we are doing the right things.

Sound easy? In principle, solution focused work seems hugely influenced by common sense and good manners, to the extent that I simply cannot believe I didn't think of it during my twenty plus years of behavioural and cognitive behavioural work. In practice however, it kind of goes against the things we are taught about how to be helpful and how to 'fix' things for people. It is weirdly difficult, for example, to prevent oneself from 'telling' other people what they ought to do to solve their problems ('What you need to do is…'). It can be difficult to sit still and listen when another person is saying they feel so hopeless they would rather be dead ('Don't say that'; 'Don't be silly'…) rather than accept that this is indeed how low the person feels. It can be hard to listen when someone says all they want is to be married or drive a car or win a million pounds when you feel certain these things are not achievable. You want to stop them wishing for what you think is impossible in order to avoid them being hurt. So solution focused principles and techniques sound easy, but might require a rewiring of some brain connections before they become second nature.

It was my co-author, Genevieve, who approached me about doing this book. It was she who put a proposal together and had the necessary correspondence with the publisher to make it a reality. I met Gen a few years ago after her mother phoned me to see if I could help because Gen was again becoming incapacitated with depression or anxiety or something that last time resulted in hospitalization and unsuccessful psychiatric treatment. Gen's journey from rocking and picking fluff off the carpet to becoming an international speaker and established author, she says, is partly due to solution focused work with me. Our respective experiences of our work together form the basis for this book.

For my part, because I was using solution focused principles, I knew within the first few minutes of meeting Gen that she was a woman of immense courage, skill, intellect and energy. Because I was looking for competencies, strengths and existing coping strategies, I immediately noticed her considerable talents and was not sidetracked by the temporary difficulties she was experiencing. My overall feeling after our first conversation was 'Wow. You can hold down a job, which you don't like, and which involves a high degree of concentration and effort, and you can maintain a relationship, a flat *and* some sort of life? How, in heavens name, do you *do* that?!' Thus, I am not in the least bit surprised at her accomplishments because the talent has been there all the time. (This is a beautiful side effect of using solution focused approaches for me. Every working day, and I do mean *every single day*, I get to meet people of such stunning qualities and abilities that my work with people who have autism, or indeed any type of 'diagnosis', is an absolute pleasure.)

Anyway, that is an introduction to the book, a bit about me, and a bit about how I met Gen. I will turn over to Gen so that she can introduce herself and set the stage for her involvement in this book.

Genevieve

How was it for me when I first met Vicky? (I have checked with Vicky in order to avoid wounding her self-esteem or professional ego so that I can say what went through my head the first time I met her.)

I came home from work that day in my usual state of having 'just coped'. Days like these were so common for me, and had been for a long time. I would finish my day depleted of everything because so much of my energy was spent trying to hold back the tears which were always there, waiting eagerly to flow if I let down my guard. More often than not I held them back well, along with the anxiety, inability to concentrate, sense of permanent doom, and disinterest in life, while at the same time trying to work out the social and emotional world using only logic and intellect. By the time I first met Vicky, I had been so eroded by this constant struggle that I had become a person who, while only in my early twenties, just didn't really enjoy life and for whom many days were spent yearning for my bed or some other place or state so I could be away from the reality of my situation.

I had become this apathetic and exhausted despite having a wonderfully supportive and loving family, supportive and well-meaning friends, and despite having been on the receiving end of attention from many mental health professionals. A multitude of different diagnoses and many attempts at 'fixing me' led me no further towards wanting to be a part of life or being able to cope without crisis after crisis. I had no reason to believe this latest intervention with this person called Vicky would be any more helpful than what had gone before.

How could a girl so well supported and loved, with so much going for her, be so inexplicably angry, depressed, anxious, distressed and unable to cope with everyday life? An eventual diagnosis of 'mild' Asperger Syndrome explained a lot. When I got the diagnosis I felt it might make sense of a life I couldn't make sense of. However, post-diagnosis, the initial euphoria which came with the understanding I thought I had found, disappeared, leaving me more desolate than ever. Thank goodness I wasn't reliant on the services offered to me and that I had the support of my family, who weren't prepared to give up on me.

At the end of her tether, my mum, desperate to find someone who could help me make sense of myself and the world around me, came across Vicky. Mum informed me that a counsellor had been found who specialized in AS and who was local to us. Mum said her name was Vicky Bliss. Vicky *Bliss*? Oh please, I thought, what a ridiculous name for a counsellor, sickening! I bet she is so perfect in every way, like a mental health Mary Poppins. I bet she never gets depressed herself, has perfect hair and make-up and wears pink. I bet she is sooo professional and thinks she has all the answers to fix me. Vomit. Nausea. Sickening. All these terms went through my head. I was so sick and tired of needing to be 'fixed'. I just wanted to live my life, for goodness sake! It can't be me who is wrong all the time, I thought. Surely, it *must* be the professionals who are getting it wrong at least some of the time. (NB if you are a mental health 'service user' don't say out loud that you think the professionals are wrong, or you'll gain another label like 'non compliant' or 'difficult to engage'. Just a tip from someone who has had that particular experience!)

If we were being problem focused we could say my attitude when hearing about Ms Bliss was cause for concern. However, if we were being solution focused we would say, despite all the apprehension I had about meeting and working with Vicky, I still, *still* agreed to the appointment and attended it on time! Good going for someone so disillusioned by 'helping professionals' eh?!

So there I was on time and Vicky came into my flat. The appointment began. Result! I thought. There was no pink in sight, no high heels, no aura of perfect professional who never gets depressed, and her hair was slightly too messy to be that of a typical professional 'fixer'. It was looking good for someone with the name 'Bliss'. What was great, too, was that normally I had to enter the 'fixer's' own space, usually an office, on their territory. Yet Vicky came to my home, my world and my territory. It was looking promising.

One thing I had grown tired of in traditional mental health settings was the fact that I had become not a person but the sum-total of my mental health notes, or my referral letter or the phone call by which I was referred. With Vicky it was different. The first things we discussed were about me as a person. Having spent so long feeling just like someone who needed to be fixed, rather than a person, I found talking about me aside from my mental health rather odd. I didn't really know what to say! We talked about things that mattered to me aside from my problems. Even in my darkest days there was something that I still had the time and energy for, and that was animals, especially horses. We talked about horses for a while before we talked about the 'problem'. Vicky too has a deep love for horses, so it felt good that I could relate to her on a level other than her being the therapist and me being the 'therapee'.

So many times I had come out of therapeutic exchanges feeling worse than when I came in; more confused and more sure of what my problems were and less sure I could ever get over them. Even the short exchange about horses, on meeting Vicky, was so important, since it helped me focus on something outside of the problem and reminded me that there were things I could do well and make sense of even if they didn't provide the answers for my getting better. I laugh sometimes that it was actually horses that got me well and not solution focused approaches, and I worry a little that I am rather a fraud to be writing about the approaches but in reality I truly don't believe that is the case.

At the end of our first session I discovered that Vicky lived very close to me and that she had two horses, Grace and Dan, that I would be welcome to meet! Wow! A therapist who isn't a typical 'professional fixer' and has horses nearby. Money well spent I reckon! I believe we had our second session of solution focused talking while grooming horses and much later, after our official therapy had ended and we began a collaboration about using solution focused approaches with people who have autism, many more solution focused conversations were had on horseback. Helpful conversations, as it turns out, don't need to be done in a 'therapy room'!

How did I start to feel better? What happens when I get depressed again? There is not a simple happy ending to my experiences with Vicky, in the sense that I met her, she cured me and I lived happily ever after. Besides, that would be too obvious, not much of a challenge and perhaps a little boring. The truth is I did get depressed again, but it was so much more short-lived; and I still have anxiety, but again, it is much better managed and does not have to become desperate. I became interested in how Vicky did what she did for me and learned more and more about solution focused approaches. The use of language, the use of existing strengths, skills and coping strategies made such sense that I wondered why I had previously been helped to focus more on my depressions, my anxiety and my inability to cope. I much preferred the discussions which highlighted those things I could continue to do well at, even when I was depressed over those discussions that underlined how bad my depression was.

Why did I want Vicky to write this guide? Quite simply I was desperate for the world to learn about what Vicky can do and the work of Vicky's consultancy, 'The Missing Link Support Services Ltd'. I promise I am not being paid by Vicky to do this, but I feel suitably qualified to be able to judge what is a good support service when I come across one because I have indeed come across many support services. When I have trained a variety of professionals in using the techniques this guide covers, Vicky and I have often questioned, 'Is it really SF approaches that work the magic or is it just Vicky? At times I have to admit I have wondered if it is just Vicky and maybe we should just be writing about 'the Bliss Technique' (blissful and magical as it sounds) rather than solution focused approaches. However, when training professionals, even if it is just the 'Bliss approach to solution focused approaches' we are teaching, when we do get professionals to role-play or assimilate these techniques into their own practice, we see time and time again that there is much more to the approach than just what Vicky can do alone. When we talk about cases where SF approaches have been successful in the life of someone with AS and we hear how others want and plan to take the lessons learnt from these examples of good practice, it makes sense to let as many people as possible learn how they can do the same, and they don't have to be 'Blissful' to do so.

More specifically about the book

So there you are. You know that Vicky is an undiagnosed autistic, solution focused psychologist in private practice, and that Gen is a solution focused survivor with AS anxious to help other people survive too. We both process information like people who have AS, we both love animals, and we both are going to try, in the course of this book, to give people ideas as to how to identify and use existing strengths to keep doing more of what works in order to feel better.

Chapter Two focuses on both the philosophy behind solution focused work and on the few techniques associated with it. It is not an extensive explanation of solution focused approaches because there are many published books and articles which explain the details of the approach quite sufficiently, and our favourites of these are listed at the end of Chapter Two. We do include a few examples to illustrate the techniques, though the dialogue is a combination of dialogues with several people with AS rather than with one individual, as it seems in the example. We tried to remain true to what happens in therapy, but in order to protect the privacy of the clients we have altered facts and woven in statements from a number of people as though they were all coming from one person, whom we have named Mike.

Chapter Three focuses on the characteristics of AS which may impact on a therapeutic relationship. We hope we show how various aspects of solution focused work fit with the strengths and needs of people with AS. This chapter is based on some of Gen's training work, so comes from the point of view of someone diagnosed with AS who also knows the benefits of solution focused work from first-hand experience. There is some background about ASD and AS, but we have not attempted a full discussion of the symptoms and diagnosis of autism because there are many publications which do this very well already. Our favourites of these are listed at the end of Chapter Three.

Chapter Four puts solution focused therapy together with people who have AS in two ways. First, a general review of Vicky's work with her Company, The Missing Link Support Services (MLSS) Ltd, during her first full year. There are not rigorously collected data to report, but there is a description of the type of work which led the MLSS to be included in a recent publication by the Department of Health (2006, p.39) as an example of good practice. The second example of solution focused brief therapy and AS is in the form of our continuing story with Mike.

Chapter Five includes solution focused approaches in everyday life. Because it has been developed as a particular way of doing therapy with people, some adjustment is required in order to use the techniques or principles outside of the therapy setting, in real life settings. We try to highlight how a solution focused approach might be adapted by employers, support workers, family members or anyone who is trying to help a person with AS use their unique personality to the full. We look at supporting someone in employment, in education, and in getting or maintaining a social life.

Chapter Six tells the stories of seven people who have AS and have experienced solution focused therapy, as well as a description of our very fun social group, the Tuesday Evening Social Club (TESC). We have changed some details of each story so that the person's privacy is protected. Where transcript information is used, we have replaced any identifying words, keeping the meaning of the exchange intact.

Finally, at the end of the book we provide some practical worksheets and resources which readers can feel free to use or amend, always quoting the source of the material, to help them reach the goals they set for themselves.

We hope this book gives some insight into solution focused approaches in general, but, more important, we want to give people both with and without ASD some practical ideas that might help them do something different when trying to have useful, positive, forward-thinking conversations with each other. We hope that readers might feel confident to try some of the ideas, and even better, to develop some ideas of their own. We would be pleased to hear from readers who have tried the approaches, and towards this end have included a contact web address in the back of the book.

Go on then… Off you go…

Chapter summary

This book is about:

- noticing and naming the strengths and skills that people with AS already use to get through their days
- developing a mutually respectful working relationship
- learning to listen to, and believe, what a person with AS says, even if you don't fully understand or agree with it
- using a common language to construct a future that is important to the person with AS
- using a common language to measure progress towards goals
- neurotypical people learning to function within, and respect, a foreign autistic culture, and vice versa.

This book is *not* about:

- supermarkets (hooray)
- assuming people with AS mean the same things as neurotypical people when they use similar language
- assuming neurotypical carers know best
- assuming there is something wrong with people who have AS
- assuming people with AS need to be more normal
- assuming people with AS need help.

Vicky's 'problem focused' assumptions

- Therapist must know how to 'fix' problems.
- People with AS want to be normal and fit in.
- Therapists should show people with AS the 'correct' way to behave.
- People with AS should 'fit in' with society in order to be happy.
- Therapist's job is to teach people with AS to identify emotions and how emotions affect behaviours and feelings, so that they can learn to behave more appropriately.

Vicky's solution focused assumptions

- People with AS are always changing regardless of anything a therapist does.
- Problems do not happen all the time; there are times when the problem is not so bad.
- People with AS are basically capable individuals who know what works for them.
- People already have the basis for positive change in the form of existing strengths and coping skills.
- People with AS have the most important point of view when it comes to setting therapeutic goals.
- Therapist's job is to notice what is already working for the person and to see how we can do more of that in order to reach the person's own goals.

Gen's observations

- SF work immediately helped her remember some strengths and skills she already had.
- Her strengths were enhanced by working with animals; SF work does not have to happen in a therapy room.

- SF work helped her to make her own sense of herself and her world.
- Vicky's 'lived-in' appearance helped Gen.
- Discussions that highlighted strengths were preferable to those that focused on depression, anxiety and her inability to cope.
- Gen's experiences of teaching people about solution focused brief therapy with people who have AS shows that ordinary professionals and carers can take the approach and do something different with it.

References

de Shazer, S., Berg, I. K., Lipchick, E., Nunnally, E. *et al.* (1986) 'Brief therapy: Focused solution development.' *Family Process 25*, 207–222.

Department of Health (2006) 'Better services for people with an autistic spectrum disorder: A note clarifying current Government policy and describing good practice.' Available at *www.dh.gov.uk/Publicationsandstatistics* (accessed 6 July 2007).

Chapter Two

Solution Focused Approaches:

Philosophy and Techniques

Introduction

Solution Focused Brief Therapy (SFBT) grew from the work of Steve de Shazer, colleagues and clients at a family practice centre in Milwaukee, USA (de Shazer *et al.* 1986). This group learned through astute listening that the people they saw in their clinic already had within themselves histories of strengths, coping skills and behaviours that were the seeds from which new solutions to present problems could grow. Accordingly, one of the central principles of SFBT is to focus more on *exceptions* to problems (that is, times when the problems aren't happening or are not as troublesome) rather than on the problem itself (de Shazer 1985). Focusing on exceptions to the problem helps both the SF therapist and the SF 'therapee' (using Gen's term from Chapter One) to notice and name the things that are already working helpfully for the person. The team combined a focus on exceptions to the problem with a belief that the client's hopes for the future were of paramount importance, and thus was born a unique type of therapy based on helping people to identify a) what they want to have in their lives and b) the existing resources which could be used to move toward those goals.

Non-problem talk

SFBT is grounded in ideas that are different from traditional problem based therapies in what we think are important ways. For example, a lot of time in SF work is spent in what is called 'non-problem' talk, which allows a person to talk about things they like and are good at while the solution focused worker listens closely for evidence of the person's skills, abilities and strengths. Time is devoted to pre-session (i.e. before the first appointment) and between-session changes as times when the person has noticed things going right. It is important to ask specifically about things that work outside of the therapy setting because these instances contain important clues about the things that are working for the client. If we know what is already working, we can make an effort to do more of that in the future.

Thus, in a session of SF therapy, one thing that stands out is the amount of time spent 'chatting' about ordinary things that are of interest to the person. This is how Gen and Vicky came to talk about horses quite early on in our therapeutic relationship, and in Chapter One Gen mentions that this was both a surprise and helpful to her. It was helpful for Vicky as well, because Gen has many competencies with regard to horses, so in listening to her talk about them, Vicky was able to collect many positive aspects to her character which we later used to help manage anxiety and depression. In more traditional approaches non-problem talking would not happen to this extent, as most of the time is spent discussing symptoms, difficulties and treatments. Non-problem talk seems tailor-made for someone with AS because of their tendency to have 'all-absorbing interests' as noted, for example, by Gillberg and Gillberg (1989). For the solution focused worker, it is an absolute gift to have a client who is willing to talk at length about their interests, because evidence of strengths and competencies will be abundant, as happened with Gen and the horses. In contrast, it can cause difficulties for a problem focused therapist to have a client who continues to talk about their own interests, because it prevents the therapist from getting on with having a fuller discussion about the problems and about what they think the client needs to do next to solve the problems. In SF work with people, it seems to be quite an unexpected treat to be encouraged to talk about a special interest rather than being asked to talk about the problems. Moreover, not only are people getting to talk about things they like, they are also being listened to by someone who is noticing quite nice things about them as they talk. People with AS often tell us this is an unusual and pleasant occurrence in their lives.

People, not problems

Non-problem talk is often one of the first things that happens when solution focused work begins, and it seems to help get the therapeutic relationship off to a good start. People expect to talk about problems or things that have gone wrong when they come to therapy, and we have noticed that eye contact, body posture, as well as the give-and-take of conversation often improves within the first 15–20 minutes of a solution focused conversation. This is all the more extraordinary when one considers that eye contact and the give-and-take of a conversation are two areas in which people with AS struggle. A worker who has developed expertise in listening will have no trouble spotting strengths during this time, as people often show evidence of strong feelings, passion, excellent memory or other cognitive skills, as well as humour, creativity and concern for other people, when they are talking about things they enjoy. We have never, ever, failed to discover and identify some positive aspects of a person's character during a first meeting, which either means people with autism are extraordinary people (which we both believe is true!) or that non-problem talk is a very good way to learn about more about *people* rather than the problem that brought them to therapy. The worker will constantly check out their observations with the person, so by the end of the first bit of work, both the worker and the person have agreed on several positive aspects of the person's character that may be applied to help reach the goals they want.

Here is an example of non-problem talk during the initial stages of a first session, after introductions and pleasantries have been taken care of:

(V – Vicky; M – Mike):

V: I know a little bit about why your social worker wanted me to see you...because she is worried about some arguments or some such thing between you and your parents. But I don't know anything about you. Tell me a bit about yourself. (*Silence*) What kinds of things do you do for fun?

M: I like old movies.

V: Yeah? What are some of your favourites?

M: I love the black-and-white ones. I like James Bond, Humphrey Bogart, Spencer Tracey. I like Laurel and Hardy too... They really make me laugh. I go to the cinema now sometimes too. There are some modern films I like but not as much as those old ones.

V: Wow. I haven't heard those old names in a while! What do you like about the old films?

M: Um...well...in a funny kind of way they are just so simple. I can't believe how life used to be. The movies make life seem so simple and black-and-white. I think I like that. Movies seem simple and predictable, kind of.

V: So you like old movies because they sometimes make you laugh, and you find them sort of simple...easy to follow?

M: Yeah. Something like that.

V: When is the best time for you to watch old movies?

M: Oh anytime... I like to read about them too.

V: Oh! So you don't just like to watch the films, you like to read about them too? What...like when they were made and things?

M: No. Not so much read about the movies, but read about the old stars. There are biographies and some autobiographies out about Bogart, Hepburn, Tracey...you know. Bogart had four wives, and the last one was Lauren Bacall...but that wasn't her real name. Her real name was Betty, but she changed it when she started starring in films. That's a funny thing to do, but a lot of movie stars do it. I don't know why exactly.

V: So you like to read factual books about movie stars?

M: Yeah. That's right. Spencer Tracey was a Catholic and married, but he and Katherine Hepburn kinda lived together too, which wasn't right. They made a lot of movies together. When Hepburn and Bogart made *African Queen* they went to Africa to do the filming. Everyone got sick but Bogart, because they all drank water but he drank only whiskey...so he didn't get sick.

V: Gosh. How do you remember all that?

M: What?... Um... I don't know... I just do. It's because I am interested in it I guess...

V: So if you are interested in something, you have a pretty good memory for the detail of it?

M: Yeah...I'd say so... I guess that's right.

V: And it sounds like you would rather work with facts than with approximations or guesses...?

M: Definitely. Yes, I like to know things. I don't understand the point of reading stories that are not true. I like things that are true.

V: So you have a good memory for things you are interested in, you like things to be simple and predictable, you like knowing how things really are – you want people to tell you the truth. Oh, and you appreciate a good laugh?

M: (*Smiling*) I guess that is so... Yeah...I like all those things.

So we have learned in a very short time that Mike has found entertainment in watching old movies and by reading facts about movie stars. We know that he prefers predictable, simple things and that he has a sense of what is the truth. We know he has a good memory, if the material is of interest to him. We might guess that he watches the films to learn more about how people behave, and to test his skills of prediction.

The worker is encouraging talk about Mike's particular interests, rather than redirecting the conversation to the arguments which prompted the referral. The worker is also checking her perceptions with Mike so that a common understanding of his strengths, competencies and perceptions can be reached. It is easy for a worker to assume that everyone with autism likes routine and predictability, but this is not actually always true. People with autism occasionally have difficulty with things that are predictable and have trouble following some kinds of routines. It is better to learn about each individual through asking questions and listening. Sometimes an entire session can be spent talking about things other than the referral problem. It turns out that this is useful, though it hardly even seems like 'therapy' in the more traditional, problem focused sense.

Leading from behind

Another important aspect of solution focused work is that the worker has no fixed idea about what the person needs to do in order to get better, nor does the worker have any fixed ideas about what the goals of the therapy should be. This means, and this is one of our absolute favourite things, that the worker comes into a session with an 'empty head' rather than a list of questions or an interview form that must be used. The worker will be experienced in asking questions designed to highlight their observations of the client's positive qualities, as well as questions to help discover the detail of what it is the person wants in the future. In that sense, the worker is leading the interaction.

The worker also has to continually check out their observations and understanding with the person to make sure they have understood a situation accurately. The worker has to be able to follow the gist of what the person thinks it is important to talk about. In this sense the worker is always one step behind in comprehension, being led in their understanding by the client.

This is born of a philosophy that people actually know what they need to do and know where they want to get to in their lives (de Shazer 1985). People, including people with autism, have already solved many, many problems, coped with many, many stresses and learned many, many new things before they meet a therapist. People come to therapy already skilled in many respects, though they may not have given much thought to how they manage the good things that they do, and the job of the therapist is to notice and name these skills so that the person has increased awareness and confidence in their own already existing abilities. Using solution focused approaches with someone who has autism is no different than with someone who does not have autism, in this respect. People with autism have no fewer skills, strengths and problem solving skills than anyone else.

Exceptions and skills

Also, SF work recognizes that people are already doing things that work, because they are surviving. Problems do not occur all of the time, so there must be some times when things are going reasonably well. As mentioned earlier (p.28), solution focused workers call these 'exceptions', and they are genuinely curious about what is happening when things are going well. The idea here is to help people notice what they are already doing that works, and then do more of that.

One of our favourite examples of how 'naturally *un*common' it is to notice success rather than notice problems comes from a news story about a school in London, though it could have been anywhere. The school had recently been inspected and found to be failing on 60 per cent of the inspection criteria. The school was put on special measures and the head teacher told the news reporter that they would have to focus on improving the 60 per cent in order to be taken off special measures. Vicky shouted at the TV 'NO! Pay attention to the 40 per cent that is going well and make sure you do more of that! The 60 per cent failure will naturally reduce if the 40 per cent compliance improves!' If the head teacher puts a spotlight on things that are not working (that is, if he focuses solely on the problems) it is quite likely that the bits of the school that *are* working will fall out of practice too, because no one is paying attention to them. That, we both feel, is rather what happens with the people we meet who have had problem focused therapy. So much time and emphasis is devoted to the problem that they (and others around them) forget about the mountain of stuff they are doing that actually works to get them through the day. So, as Gen notes in Chapter One, even though she had reservations about how useful Vicky could be, she still agreed to give her a try and was on time for the appointment. How did she *do* that?! Already there are important skills and attitudes in evidence.

The process of beginning to identify existing strengths of the person begins, as we have seen, with non-problem talk. Below is an example of continuing the job of noticing and naming skills by seeking exceptions to the referral problem. We continue with Mike's story:

V: Mike, the social worker is worried about some argument that you must've had with your parents.

M: (*Looks at his shoes*)

V: Well...what I want to know is, how did you get the argument to stop?

M: (*Looks up*) Well. I don't know really. (*Long silence*)

V: (*More silence*)

M: Um. I think I must've walked out of the room.

V: Heck...well done you! How did you know to do that?

M: Well. I don't know. I didn't think about what to do, I just wanted to get away from them because they were making me mad. I might have slammed the door when I left... I was so mad.

V: Do you think you handled that in the best way you could?

M: Yeah. Yeah, probably I did. Because before I would actually pick up stuff to throw, but this time I just walked out.

V: Wow. So this last argument was a bit better than others?

M: I wouldn't say it was better. Better would be if they didn't happen at all wouldn't it? My dad hates it when I walk away too. That makes him madder but I don't know what else to do. He follows me and that makes me madder and then the argument just keep going. They pick on me all the time and they think I can't do anything right.

V: So...did you argue today...before coming here?

M: What? No.

V: Gosh...so even though they pick on you all the time, you didn't argue today? How did you manage to be picked on and not argue?

M: Well...well...they didn't say anything about how I was dressed or what I ate for breakfast. Oh wait. Yes. Mum did say I should have eaten something else for breakfast. But I didn't say anything back.

V: Ah...so sometimes you can be picked on and not start an argument? What a skill. How do you do that?

M: Um...I don't know. I guess sometimes I just ignore it.

So it turns out that Mike has quite a few skills and strategies he is already using, but it sounds like he has not thought much about these. Putting words to the excellent coping skills he has will make him more likely to do them again in the future. This also contributes to an increase in self-esteem because we are finding skills that he already has as part of his lovely nature. It quickly becomes clear in these kinds of conversations that Mike is much more than a summary or a product of the problems that brought him to see me.

Frequently a lack of attention to the existing skills of someone with AS is particularly evident when carers are focused on 'normalizing' the person, or on 'getting them to see sense'. A person with AS may *not* want to fit in with the non-autistic community all the time, and likely as not they will already have tried to fit in, without a great deal of success. SF work does not accommodate therapists who want to work to their own agenda of what they think would be best for their client.

In order for solution focused approaches to work, the therapist needs to be confident enough to really believe that the person knows what is best for them, even when the therapist doesn't agree with what they say. In the example above, Mike says his parents pick on him all the time. A problem focused therapist might be tempted to try and talk him out of this by saying something like 'Surely they don't pick on you *all* the time?' which sets the therapist and Mike up on opposing sides of the desk.

Believing what clients say does have the potential to cause some ethical dilemmas, though to date (in six years of solution focused work) no dilemmas have arisen that the client and Vicky haven't been able to solution-focus their way out of!

Some examples of ethical dilemmas which have arisen are when the person with AS has insisted that he does not have a problem, and that everyone else will have to change in order for him to stop being aggressive. During the course of conversation, it was Vicky's opinion (though she tried to suppress it) that this particular client did indeed have a very rigid way of processing information that was leading him to become more suspicious and angry than was strictly necessary. Yet he did not agree that he contributed to his difficulties with other people, so Vicky had to bend around the language and beliefs of this man in order to work with him to achieve *his* goals, rather than goals she would have liked to set for him.

Another man said that he would know Vicky had done a good job of working with him when he had a wife, a house and some children. If we could achieve this during our time together, he thought, his problems would be solved. Vicky swallowed a 'Yikes!' that nearly escaped out of her mouth, and suggested that was quite a tall order, and that it fell somewhere outside the remit of what she had been hired to do. However, in keeping with what this fella wanted, they talked about what he thought would be better when he had a wife, and found that some of those small improvements were within the remit of the therapy.

In another example, a young woman was frequently having her food and money stolen by people claiming to be her friends. This happened when she got a flat instead of living on the street. Her 'mates' knew her from when she lived on the street, and she said that them stealing from her was not a problem for her, because it was just the way things were on the street. She said that when she was homeless she did the same thing. Vicky as the worker wanted to help her not be stolen from, when all along the client was not worried at all about this state of affairs.

Empty-headed and curious

A solution focused worker is curious about the person's preferred future; that is, what would an ordinary day without the problems be like? People come to therapy because either they, or someone else, want something to change, but without specific questioning they probably have not thought through the detail of exactly what they would like to be different, and what is already happening that they would like to keep, in their lives. An empty-headed therapist is one who has space to take on board the unique details from the individual about what will be different when their problems have gone away.

Part of the therapist having an 'empty head' extends to this aspect of the work because the therapist does not set goals for the client, or come into a session with any ideas about what might be best for the person, or what answers are the 'right' ones to give in any case. The therapist gives up her fixed beliefs about what clients need to do in order to get better. In this sense, the therapist does not have to have extensive knowledge of the various schools of thought, such as CBT, psychoanalysis, applied behaviour analysis, or similar. What they need in place of this theoretical knowledge is a genuine belief that the person with AS already has strengths and skills, knows where they want to get to, and that these two things can be effectively matched up.

Instead of already knowing how to fix things, the worker will be skilled at helping the person imagine the future they want, plus noticing the details of what will be different when that future is attained. It is lovely, as sometimes happens, when the therapist and client jointly notice that little bits of the preferred future are already happening. This gives a nice boost of hope and confidence to the person and sets the stage for even more little bits of the preferred future to start being noticed.

The curiosity of the therapist is genuine, and requires very well developed ears. Not big ones necessarily, but ears that are attuned to hearing strengths and clues as to how the person is going to move forward. The therapist no longer has a crutch in the form of fixed ideas about what the client needs to do in order to 'get better', so they need to listen like a demon so that they can, with the client, formulate a reasonable way forward.

It would take a miracle

de Shazer and his colleagues noticed that some people could talk about their preferred future more easily if they thought about just an ordinary day without the problems (de Shazer 1988). One of the techniques for helping a person think about the details of an ordinary day without the problems that brought them to therapy is called 'the Miracle Question' (de Shazer 1988). The text of the Miracle Question is as follows:

> Suppose that one night while you were asleep, there was a miracle and this problem was solved. How would you know? What would be different?
>
> (de Shazer 1988, p.5)

People familiar with the characteristics of someone with autism will immediately spot several difficulties with this question; however, Gen and Vicky thought it worth including the original text of the question so that we are clear about any changes that we make in practice. Some of the difficulties with this question for people with AS include the use of imagination, the literal interpretation of the word 'miracle', having to pretend problems disappear, and thinking about things being different than they are right in the moment. It is worth noting that these same difficulties also sometimes occur with people who do not have autism.

An example of one way the text of the Miracle Question was adapted to suit Mike's situation with good results follows:

V: So Mike...if tonight when you went to sleep...your dad had a personality transplant that made him the best dad ever...but you didn't know this happened because you were asleep...what would be the first thing you would notice about your dad in the morning that told you something was different about him?

M: Ha. I don't think that could happen.

V: No, I know it doesn't fit with your logical, practical, truthful personality! But it might give us some good information. Go on...what would you notice?

M: Don't know.

V: Well...would you get up at the same time, if you had the best dad in the world?

M: Yeah...yeah...that wouldn't change.

V: Would you get dressed and washed just the same?

M: Yeah...I guess so... I would still have breakfast by myself though.

V: OK...so what would be the first thing that would tell you your dad had changed?

M: Well...maybe we could just ride our bikes around the streets instead of going to the gym and riding on those bikes that don't actually go anywhere. That would be better. I would still get exercise, which is what he wants, but I wouldn't be sweating in that stinky gym.

V: So part of what you would like to happen is that you and Dad find more 'natural' ways to exercise instead of going to the gym?

It is very possible we would not have reached this level of detail if it weren't for a version of the Miracle Question, and if it weren't for the therapist's persistence in pursuing an answer to the question, even though it initially seemed as though Mike struggled to think up an answer.

There are other, slightly more concrete questions that solution focused workers might ask to help a person think through what they want to be different in their lives. These are simpler questions, such as 'What will be happening when you know you do not need to see me any more?' Or, 'How will you know that our time together has been well spent today?' Or, 'What will you notice about yourself when you are getting better? What will other people notice?' Or, 'If you and I work really well together, what will you notice that tells you we have done the right things?' The task of the worker here is to look for details of what will be different when things are going well, and to keep checking their understanding of these differences with the person.

We think the important part of these preferred future questions involves the person identifying the detail of how they want things to be. A solution focused worker will develop expertise in asking questions designed to elicit specific details of what the person will notice as things get better. The more descriptive the detail, the easier it will be for the person and those around them to notice when those things start to happen.

Language and listening

A solution focused worker will be an expert at paying attention to language, in terms both of the language they themselves use, and of the language preferred by the person. People have told us that one of the ways they know we are listening to them is because we use their own language back to them. It seems important for the worker to be able to pick up on the terms used by the person and to adjust their own language to suit that of the person.

The language used by the worker will convey hope and the expectation that positive changes will occur – indeed, have already occurred. The worker will also use language to rephrase things the person has said, for example:

> *M*: I don't think things will ever change.
>
> *V*: Right now, you think things are pretty much stuck. Is that right?

By using 'right now' the therapist introduces the idea that Mike's expressed feeling of 'stuckness' is temporary, suggesting the possibility that this position can change. The therapist also carefully repeats the word 'think' because that is the word that Mike has used. Alternative words might have been 'believe', 'feel', 'see' or 'know', but as Mike used 'think', so too does the therapist. By adding 'Is that right?' on the end the worker is checking that their rephrasing, and introduction of the word 'stuck', seems right to Mike. These may seem minor points, but the worker's skill in this area is important to helping the person get to where they want to be.

We have already banged on a bit about the importance of the therapist being a good listener. In solution focused work, the resources and aims that the client brings are the main tools with which the therapist has to work. If the therapist doesn't listen well, she is left with no tools! And a therapist with no tools is not a pretty sight.

The idea of professionals not listening to people with AS is not new to us. People who have AS report to both Gen and Vicky that they are not used to being listened to by therapists and workers! As part of routine feedback on the service, when asked to comment about what they like about solution focused work, people with AS noted that Vicky really listened to them and that made a difference. Individual comments included one by a particularly astute man who said, 'Other therapists only half listened, then they filled in the other half with what they thought was right. Vicky didn't do this. She listened one hundred per cent.' Another individual said, 'I could tell Vicky was listening because she used my own words back to me,' and still another said, 'I felt listened to and I think that in itself was enough to make me feel better.' What a simple yet effective intervention that was!

On the topic of being listened to, Gen writes:

> I couldn't agree more with the astute man's comment about being half listened to. Often when I speak to service users and those in autism services who really 'get it' the sentiment is the same. Whether it be based on exchanges with a therapist, a support worker or a service manager, rarely do those with autism get listened to, not half listened to, but 'really' listened to. I used to believe that this was just laziness, a lack of effort or will on the part of these poor listeners. However, now, although I believe these issues still play a part for the non-listeners, I have begun to learn that perhaps this may be more of a struggle for them than I realised. I have come to learn that perhaps this has got something to do with the difference in being neurotypical or autistic, and that 'really listening' is as difficult for those without autism as for with those with autism, and vice versa. From this point of view, I feel it may be an issue of admitting this inability and (horror of horrors) admitting that one (a therapist for

> example) is not as all-knowing as was once thought, and maybe even not as competent as necessary when it comes to working well with individuals who have autism.

Gen goes on to say:

> One thing I found so helpful from Vicky was her stance of 'not knowing'. I have to admit at first when I met Vicky, having met therapists who probably put all their energy into 'having the answers' and 'looking professional', that I was somewhat suspicious and disconcerted. I admit to suspecting that Vicky didn't really know what she was doing and was unprofessional. (*Cue snorts of laughter from Vicky...*) However, having been faced with this 'unprofessional not-knower' I was delighted to discover, over time, that this was what I had been looking for. The sensation of being 'really listened' to, for me, meant someone who really could use my language and work with my way of seeing the world, rather than sticking with their own view of the world.

People with AS usually know what they are talking about, and a therapist's or worker's job is made so much easier by showing genuine curiosity, listening well and believing what clients say (and perhaps lying down until one's own preconceived ideas of 'autism', 'right' and 'wrong' pass into oblivion).

Who's got the power?

People with AS are often very used to being told by people without AS what they should and should not do, or what is right and what is wrong. They are used to other folks not understanding or even asking their opinions on things or the reasons behind their behaviours. The issue of power imbalance between worker and client seems particularly important in work with someone who has AS, because they are already in a devalued, minority position within society. We find that frequently people with AS have difficulty cooperating with workers who behave as though they have power over them by telling them what to do or only half listening to them.

Many people with AS are unable to cooperate with instructions that do not make sense to them, so when people say such things as 'You can't do that', or 'You must do it this way', clients may naturally rebel without seeing the broader picture. solution focused work does not result in the therapist having the power to tell the individual what they need to do, which comes as a nice surprise to people with AS.

The exchange between worker and client is meant to be on an 'expert to expert' basis, so that each person shares equal responsibility for coming to a common understanding of the way forward. A solution focused worker would pay attention to issues of power, and would seek to minimise the imbalance of power that naturally exists between client and worker. Many individuals with AS also have a very strong sense of social justice and may have a drive to be on an equal footing (just like 'normal' people!) where possible. What a joy it is, therefore, when using solution focused approaches, that people with AS can have an equal footing where their own expertise is worth as much, if not more, than the expertise of the therapist, who by virtue of this standing does not have all the answers.

We think this is a sensible and critical aspect of working with people who have autism, because they have built a unique understanding of themselves and of their world which has helped them to survive thus far. It makes sense from our point of view for the therapist to be the one to be flexible in his or her ability to quickly learn the language and points of reference of the person, rather than expect the person with AS to quickly learn the language and points of reference of the therapist. More traditional therapists seem to require that the person learn how to 'correctly' use the language of emotions, for example, whereas in solution focused work it is the therapist who is required to learn the person's language. One can see how important it is for the solution focused worker to be able to use the person's unique language and frames of reference in order to understand what it is the person wants to achieve. We continue with Mike:

V: So...you want to stop arguing with your mum and dad?

M: No. Really what I want is for them to stop picking on everything I say or do.

V: Ah. Do they know that they pick on you?

M: Yes...how could they not know? They are pretty stupid if they don't know that, aren't they? They say they don't but they know they do.

V: Huh. So you ask them not to pick on you and they say they are not picking on you?

M: Yes. That makes me so mad. They pick on everything.

V: What's the last thing they picked on you about?

M: Well...this morning...Mum told me I should have eaten something else for breakfast...fruit or something...cereal wasn't enough. She thinks I am stupid...that I don't know when I've had enough to eat...

V: Oh, I see. Mum picks on you when she is worried that you haven't had enough to eat? Could she be worried rather than think you are stupid? It is a mum's job to worry... They do it rather a lot.

M: Well...yes, she does say she worries...

V: So picking on you might be her way of worrying about you?

In this context, it is important to stick with Mike's perception of being 'picked on' even though his parents do not agree that this is what they are doing. In his frame of reference, he is being picked on. Through careful use of language, being picked on (which is seen as a negative thing) is paired with being worried about (which is seen as a characteristic of Mum, and a possibly nice characteristic at that). The possibility is that some of the anger about being picked on might naturally be dissipated through an understanding of Mum's motivations.

Scaling

Scales are another technique used by solution focused workers. Typically, this involves rating something on a scale of 0–10, where 0 represents the worst something can be and 10 represents the best something can be. As with the Miracle Question, people experienced in the field of autism will immediately see some difficulties with this technique, in as much as it involves using abstract concepts, such as 'better than/worse than', and abstract thinking is often not a strong skill for people with autism. Also, the ability to make a cognitive connection between 'a lot of confidence' and the number 10, for example, may be difficult for someone with AS. Indeed, it has been known to be difficult for some people *without* autism too.

The intent of this technique is to provide a bridge to a common understanding between the therapist and the person. For example, if a common understanding of what will be happening when the person rates themselves at a seven can be achieved with the worker, then detailed discussions can also be had about where the person rates themselves now and, perhaps even more important, what the next number up on the scale will look like. This allows kind of a shorthand conversation to develop that tells both the person with AS and the worker what the next little signs of successful work will be. Mike helps us out again with an example:

V: So, Mike, if ten represents the best parents in the world and zero represents the worst parents in the world, where would you rate your parents now?

M: Um...I don't even know what the best parents in the world would look like! Um...well, they are not the worst because I know parents that are far worse than mine. I would say they are about a four.

V: A four! What makes them a four?

M: Well...like you say, they do worry about me and I know they want things to be better for me, and sometimes they don't pick on me about things.

V: Wow. That's good (*Vicky has an option here to follow up on these lovely exceptions or to carry on with the scaling.*) If ten is the best...what number would be 'good enough' for you?

M: A ten of course! I want the best! (*Chuckles*) Um, an eight maybe.

V: OK...and if you are on four now, what will have happened when you move that rating up to a five?

M: Oh...if I go home tonight and don't feel like they are picking on me, then that will be a good thing.

V: And if ten is complete confidence and zero is no confidence at all, how confident are you that you won't be picked on when you go home?

M: Oh...now you're asking...a...seven.

V: Seven! Yahoo! That's very confident! What gives you such confidence?!

So in this example, scales are used both for indicating a 'good' parent and for confidence in Mike's stated aim. As often happens, a secondary gain of using scales is more clarity in the aims of the work. In Mike's case, he decided that if *he felt* they weren't picking on him he would feel better, whereas before he wanted them to *actually* not pick on him. The worker's attention to language use would be important to highlight this difference to him.

Vicky has used some visual aids to help some clients, and the concepts can be varied a little bit in an effort to make the idea of scales more accessible to those who have difficulty with the numerical ratings. For example, use a little square to represent 'a little happy' and a big square to represent 'a lot happy – like when getting presents on your birthday', and ask the person to point to which square seems to fit with their mood at the time. Likewise, simple cartoon faces can be drawn to suggest different possible ratings. Once some type of rating can be given, very interesting and enlightening discussions can be held, where the person with AS teaches the worker how they manage to get from 'little happy' to 'big happy' on an ordinary day. Within that discussion, the worker will be able to hear many useful things about coping skills, points of reference, and about what is important to that person.

When we have asked workers (such as direct care staff, social workers, nurses etc.) to rate, on the scale of 0–10, their level of confidence that the person with AS will actually attain the goals they want, we often get an apologetic 'five' or lower. (Remember that smaller numbers on this scale represent little confidence and larger numbers represent lots of confidence.) It is as if the workers believe they ought to have more confidence or that a rating of 'ten' is the 'right' answer. The good news is that there are no bad answers to a scaling question! Workers are as delighted with a 'two' as with an 'eight' because the point of the answer is to help us understand more about where the person is at, and what the next step might be. We want to know 'Why a five instead of a four?' This helps the worker to identify all the positive aspects of the situation which give the person even a little bit of confidence. Then we want to know, 'What will have happened when you rate your confidence one step higher, at a five?' and this tells us what the person will be looking for in the near future. Other possible questions include, 'What number on the scale will be good enough?' because people are not always looking to rate themselves at a ten, and it is good to check this out rather than assume we know where people want to be.

Solution focused work and autism – a match we seriously think was made in heaven. The person needing to be most flexible is the therapist, and the person who knows most about what helps them get what they want is the client. This is playing toward the natural strengths of both individuals.

Summary

Solution focused work has two main aims:

1. to identify what clients want in their lives (their goals)
2. to identify existing resources that can be used to achieve these goals.

The philosophy of SF work includes:

- therapists learning a lot about the person and only a little about the problem
- therapists leading the therapy from one step behind the client
- identifying existing strengths, skills and hopes for the future
- therapists being genuinely curious and 'empty-headed'
- therapists developing a common language and working on an expert to expert basis with the client.

The techniques of SF work include:

- noticing pre-session and between-session changes
- non-problem talk
- coping questions
- seeking exceptions
- learning about preferred futures (maybe the Miracle Question)
- scaling questions.

References

de Shazer, S. (1985) *Keys to Solutions.* New York: W.W. Norton & Company.

de Shazer, S., (1988) *Clues: Investigating Solutions in Brief Therapy.* New York: W.W. Norton & Company.

de Shazer, S., Berg, I. K., Lipchik, E., Nunnally, E. *et al.* (1986) 'Brief therapy: Focused solution development.' *Family Process 25*, 207–221.

Gillberg, I. and Gillberg, C. (1989) 'Asperger syndrome: Some epidemiological considerations.' *Journal of Child Psychology and Psychiatry 33*, 813–842.

Recommended reading

George, E., Iveson, C. and Ratner, H. (1990) *Problem to Solution: Brief Therapy with Individuals and Families.* London: BT Press.

Gingerich, W. (2000) 'SFBT: A review of outcome research.' *Family Process 39*, 477–498.

Iveson, C. (2002) 'Solution focused brief therapy.' *Advances in Psychiatric Treatment 8*, 149–157.

McKeel, A.J. (1999) as discussed in A.J. Macdonald (2003) 'Research in Solution-Focused Brief Therapy' in B. O'Connell and S. Palmer (eds) *Handbook of Solution-Focused Therapy.* London: Sage Publications.

O'Connell, B. (2005) *Solution-Focused Therapy* (second edition). London: Sage Publications.

Chapter Three

Autistic Characteristics and Solution Focused Therapy

Introduction

As with the previous chapter, this chapter is not intended as a full discussion of the condition known as Autistic Spectrum Disorder (ASD), a subset of which is Asperger Syndrome (AS). This chapter aims to give the reader an overview of the characteristics of a person with AS, with special attention to how those characteristics may affect the process of therapy. Our overview, presented here, comes from our experience both as people having characteristics of autism and as people working with other autistic people and their families. For readers who would like to know more, there are many books written about autism, and we have listed some of our favourites at the end of this chapter.

There have been many attempts to describe the characteristics of people who have autism, mainly driven by a medical model of listing symptoms, rating the symptom severity and arriving at a diagnosis. In the early days (the terms 'early infantile autism' and 'autistic psychopathy' were first used in the 1940s to describe people with autism and AS respectively) attention was focused on people who fit neither the criteria of established abnormal behaviour (i.e. diagnosable mental illness), nor within the limits of 'normal' behaviour. The view was that people who had autism or AS 'suffered' from this 'disorder' of development and that they were as such 'mentally handicapped'

(Bogdashina 2006, p.21). Oh dear. Thankfully views and the humans who have them have evolved over time and it is now recognized that people can have autism in the form of AS, without being 'mentally handicapped'. Indeed many people with AS have above average abilities to learn and use new information.

As is often the case in science, many professionals discussed, agreed and disagreed about the existence of autism, and the first diagnostic criteria were not developed until 1989 (Gillberg and Gillberg 1989). It was a few years later that diagnostic criteria were established for AS as something separate from autism (World Health Organisation 1990; American Psychiatric Association 1994).

Autism is now generally accepted to be a spectrum disorder, although we prefer the word 'difference' to 'disorder'. On one end of the spectrum a person with severe autism will have a significant learning disability and may not use spoken language at all. Some of their disabilities are obvious for people to see, which in one way makes it easier for them to receive support. To date, these individuals need a high degree of support and would not usually be referred for a talking type of therapy. (Carers for these individuals, however, may be helped considerably by a solution focused approach!)

On the other end of the spectrum are individuals who have above average intelligence and do not appear to have disabilities. It is at this end of the spectrum that AS falls. People with AS may have jobs, partners or children and may appear to be successful in some respects. Their social life, however, is likely to be characterised by few friends and they are likely to be considered 'odd' in some ways by people who know them well.

By any historical standard then, autism is a relatively new 'disability' (again we would say 'difference' rather than 'disability') to have, for professionals to recognize, let alone to treat, and for society to tolerate. It is most often considered a 'disability' by professionals, though we hope the tide is slowing turning so that the views of people who have AS may start to prevail. This would mean, as we have noted earlier, AS and autism in general would be seen as a 'difference' rather than a disability.

There are starting to be professional references to support a social-disability-but-a-personal-difference view in the literature now. For example, Beardon (in press) states (speaking about people with autism):

> I would say that the only reason we use the term 'disorder' is because there are more NT people ('neurotypical' or people without autism) than there are people with autism. What we should be talking about is

> difference, not disorder; we should be recognising that just because a person with autism develops differently it is not automatically a negative state (i.e. 'disorder') but a difference that needs acknowledgement.

Gen follows this up with a comment about the social model of disability by suggesting that autism is a difference which is only disabling when in the company of inflexible, intolerant, and uninformed neurotypical people.

So, for example, if a person with AS is in employment, but his colleagues and boss do not understand the reasonable adjustments which could be made to help him work better, the person with AS is disabled by work colleagues rather than by the AS. It's a subtle but important difference.

Autism treatment history

The medically oriented professions in the late 1980s and 1990s sought to develop comprehensive treatments by listing each difficulty shown by a person with autism and then working out how to 'get rid of' or moderate the effect of each symptom. Early on (in the 1940s and for pretty much the five decades following) people with autism, at least those who also had learning disabilities, were seen as people needing to be 'fixed' or 'normalized' (e.g. Wolfensburger 2000) by expert professionals. The fixing was mainly attempted by trying to help people with autism (and learning disabilities) become more 'normal' (and, one might argue, less individual).

Within recent years, people with autism have been writing books which have captured the attention of a handful of professionals (e.g. Grandin 1996; Williams 1996) and there is beginning to be a slow turn from seeing autism as a collection of undesirable characteristics equalling a 'disability' to seeing people who have autism as people who process information in a different, but not necessarily a disabled, way. This philosophy about 'disability' takes a social constructionist view (which also underpins solution focused work) and would say, as Gen says, that people with autism are indeed disabled, but by the society which refuses to accept and enjoy their differences rather than by their own internal autistic characteristics (e.g. Malloy and Vasil 2002).

According to prevalence research, which has inherent difficulties even when conducted rigorously, the numbers of people with autism have been rising since the early 1940s, when it was considered a rare disorder. The developing estimate of the number of people affected by autism was about four or five out of every 10,000 births. More recently, this estimate has risen to about 120–130 per 10,000 births (Kadesjo, Gillberg and Hagberg 1999). This has prompted a debate (professionals *love* debates) over whether or not this is due to an increased awareness of the 'condition', a broadening of the diagnostic criteria, or due genuinely to an increasing number of people who have the 'condition'. If it is the latter, of course, science would want to know why this is so (Bogdashina 2006).

No matter which outcome is agreed after the debate, the increase in people acquiring the diagnosis of autism puts pressure on services to create useful supports for this growing group of people. Solution focused work, we know from our experience, usually provides an excellent basis for providing the support needed. Focusing on the considerable strengths and skills of a person with AS often (though of course not always) seems to result in increased self-esteem, increased movement towards goals, and calmer behaviour. Even better, these results seem to be forthcoming for many carers as well.

Understanding autism the professional way

The characteristics of someone who has autism have been placed by professionals into three categories:

1. difficulty making and maintain social relationships
2. difficulty in communication
3. an impairment of imagination.

These three areas have come to be known as the 'triad of impairments' (Wing 1992). Each category is assessed for presence or absence by behavioural indicators which can be seen or reported. There is a caveat that the difficulties must be present throughout the person's life, as AS is considered to be a pervasive developmental disorder.

Worryingly, as discussed by Ghaziuddin (2005), the behavioural indicators of autism can appear similar to other kinds of diagnostic conditions such as obsessive-compulsive disorder, schizophrenia, and bipolar disorder, among others, and people with true AS can thus slip quietly into non-specialist mental health services for support. There *are* differences between autism and these other disorders but they can be difficult to spot, especially if the professionals involved do not have experience with autism. As a case in point, a person who had been diagnosed with AS was recently told by a clinical psychologist that autism was not possible to diagnose because the condition was not described well enough to be assessed. To you, sir, we say, 'Rubbish – buy this book or one of hundreds of others and get up to date before you really do some damage.'

Understanding autism the autistic way

In contrast to the professional, medically oriented view, at least one writer with autism (Grandin 1996) has expressed her differences as a triad of information-processing problems (storing, organizing and retrieving information), cognitive differences (applying information and seeing 'bits' rather than 'the whole') and sensory/perceptual differences (experiencing things differently), which puts rather a different light on the way one thinks of autism. She, and, we think, other people with autism, emphasize the neurological and biological differences within the person, whereas the professionals responsible for diagnosing autism place emphasis on the outward, observable symptoms of autism. So Grandin might say that a person with autism who covers his ears and rocks in a nightclub would be doing so because his sensory experience is different than that of those around him. He is likely to experience the noises as painful rather than pleasant. A professional, on the other hand, might say that the person was showing this behaviour because they are 'autistic'. The former sounds, we think, like someone who can be helped, while the latter sounds like someone who has a disability with no cure.

Along similar lines, one of the things we feel strongly about is that professionals should not dismiss any very real mental health issues faced by an AS person as 'not treatable' because they are part of the autism. In other words, people with AS have mental health problems just like people without AS, and ought to have access to the same sorts of help. We also recognize, however, that workers in mental health services need to learn how to work with people who process information in the way that people with autism do.

In the remainder of this chapter, we look at how characteristics of someone with AS might affect the process of both problem focused and solution focused therapy.

So what help is available?

People with AS of course have mental health needs, and according to research appear much more likely to suffer mental health problems than their non-autistic peers (Deudney 2004; Ghaziuddin 2005). There is a sense of difference, confusion, anxiety and isolation common to many people with AS, and according to our own experiences, as well as the National Autistic Society in the UK (2001), there is little in terms of effective therapy or support that is available for this group. The NHS report provides statistics showing that over half of the adults on whom their report was based suffered some form of mental health problem, and yet very few individuals had access to appropriate support for their mental health issues (National Autistic Society 2001).

In the main, the therapeutic support that is available to people with AS (and people without AS often enough) is problem focused and/or medication based. This support comes under such titles as cognitive behavioural therapy (CBT), interpersonal therapy (IPT), psychodynamic psychotherapy, and even person centred therapy. These are therapies that are recommended by the National Institute of Clinical Excellence (2007) for people who suffer from mental health difficulties. Their guidance recommends primarily CBT, and as a consequence, this is the type of therapy most frequently taught to professionals and offered to clients. NICE guidance is driven by research, you see, and CBT has been more widely researched than SFBT. The difficulty with research is that it doesn't very often mirror real life. The NICE guidelines also do not give advice for people with AS who experience mental health difficulties.

Much of what is available in terms of treatment is given by professionals without specific knowledge of autism, or by professionals without the ability to apply such knowledge as is available without superimposing their own values and views of acceptable behaviour onto those of the client. Consequently they may compound the different-ness, confusion, anxiety and isolation that people with AS often feel. Genevieve recalls experiencing CBT, along with other problem focused therapies, prior to receiving SFBT. She says:

> I was a diligent client. I did every scrap of homework, asked questions and worked hard at understanding what the therapist was trying to say. Somehow it was all not related to me though. It seemed to relate more to the way the therapist maybe viewed the world, or this 'average' or 'typical' person I didn't feel I related to. I spent more time trying to work out how a 'typical' person might see the situation than I ever did working out how the therapy might help me. I could understand the concepts academically, but I could not apply this understanding to my situation. I ended up feeling inadequate yet again, despite the therapist's best attempts to help and despite my own attempts to make the therapy work. I came to realise, having received this and similar therapies, that the idea that any therapist or support professional should feel consciously or subconsciously that they had the 'answers' or the capacity to fix anyone was absurd. No wonder therapy wasn't working for me.

Gen further writes:

> I used to be so hopeful between sessions, whether they were sessions with a psychiatrist or counsellor, as though in the time between them I just had to wait. I had become dependent on them to give me answers. I knew deep down I was searching for someone who could help me find my own answers, yet I carried on. I used to ask them direct questions about what I ought to be doing and I was always faced with the maddening answer of 'I can't advise you.' This frustrated me because, as a person who largely navigates the social and emotional world through logic and facts, what I meant in my language by 'I want you to advise me' was 'I want you to advise me how to make sense of this therapy/support, etc. in a way that makes sense to me as a person, not to you as a therapist or person trained in therapeutic discourses.'

This was one example of when the only thing the therapist knew to do was not effective for the client. If that therapist had been able to ask questions designed to notice and name some of the things that had already worked for Gen, together they might have been able to set the CBT model aside and move on to using Gen's own theory of change in order to help her do 'more of what works'. Let's move on to look more specifically at some of the differences people with AS bring to therapy.

Therapy and social interaction differences

It's all in the face

People with autism sometimes do funny things with their eyes. It is difficult for some people with AS to process information from several sources at one time. So, for example, if they are trying to think while they are talking, they may avert their eyes from another person in order to minimise the amount of information coming to them. Likewise, while they are listening to someone else talk, they may avert their eyes in order to focus their concentration on what they are hearing, without being distracted by the considerable visual information coming to them from the person's face. To an untrained worker, this makes the person with autism appear suspicious, ignorant or 'too weird'. Therapists sometimes fall into this trap and mistake unusual eye contact for avoidance of important issues or denial of what the therapist is saying. They even sometimes think the person with AS is not listening because they do not have good eye contact. Some well-meaning but misguided workers may even try to get the AS person to increase their eye contact in order to appear more normal, without discussing the cost/benefit for the person with AS.

Another difficulty with not looking at a speaker, of course, is that people will miss nonverbal cues from the speaker's face or body that would help them to better understand what is being said. Neurotypical workers sometimes do not know that only the verbal part of their message is being received when they are working with a person who has poor eye contact. They may later be surprised to learn that the person didn't understand the way in which they said the information because the AS person didn't see the raised eyebrows or the smile on the speaker's face.

On the other hand, people with autism might stare too intensely at someone. Sometimes they get 'stuck' if they are looking at a person when they begin processing mental or auditory information. Their energies and attention get diverted to the processing they are doing, and they forget that their eyes are locked onto a person in a kind of maniacal way. Again, to the untrained worker, this may signal ignorance, weirdness or an attempt to intimidate the other person. If the worker behaves in accordance with these beliefs without checking them out, the person with autism is likely to be confused and astounded to learn that the worker perceived them as being intimidating when this was never, ever an intention of theirs.

One can see how big a problem this could be, for example, if a psychiatrist, untrained in AS, interpreted intense eye contact as the patient trying to be intimidating, when in reality the person was simply unaware of the effect their eyes were having on the psychiatrist. We think errors of interpretation in this way may be a common beginning to a misdiagnosis and inappropriate treatment.

People with AS often do not use the typical range of facial expressions to enhance their communication. They often do not smile purely for social reasons, such as when greeting people. A worker may not be able to rely on a person's face to tell if they are feeling guilty, worried, anxious, sad or happy, as the person's face may look pretty much the same in each instance. In a therapeutic setting, a person with AS may not smile when they meet the therapist, or even during therapy, which can make a therapist feel disheartened or unappreciated.

Again, erroneous conclusions may be reached by the therapist, such as, the client is depressed, not 'in touch' with their feelings, denying their emotions, unable to establish relationships, or any number of similar conclusions. Therefore, it is ever so important that the therapist voice their suspicions and check these out with the person. Of course, it goes without saying by now that if a therapist is asking the client for feedback on one of their assumptions, they need to believe the client when they respond.

Relationships

Autism is a pervasive developmental difference, which means there has to have been evidence of significant differences from a very early age. People with AS are likely to tell of a childhood spent with perhaps one or two close friends with whom they watched other children from the edge of groups.

Frequently there is reported a lack of pretend play in which the ideas of the AS person were incorporated along with the ideas of other children. In fact, people with AS are likely to report minimal interest in joining in with other children, though they may be fascinated to watch other children in an attempt to work out the rules by which these (seemingly) illogical children play. If asked to join in, some children with AS will happily try to do so, but more likely they will not wish to join in until they feel secure in their knowledge of the 'rules' of the game. This tendency may follow them into adulthood, when if asked to participate in therapy, they may be very quiet and appear withdrawn while they work out the rules and context of the therapeutic situation.

Also, children with AS often prefer parallel play, where they can do their own running or jumping independently of whatever the rest of the group are doing. They may struggle more with cooperative play, where there are rules which they do not yet grasp. The overall picture of a child with AS is one of poor or delayed integration with people of the same age.

The worker may notice that an AS adult in therapy seems reluctant to 'fully engage' with the therapist, preferring to maintain a good intellectual/emotional distance from the therapist until they can work out a context in which to process information about the person. Much like odd eye contact, this can make a worker think all sorts of things, such as the client is 'resistant to change', unable to form a therapeutic relationship, and so on. Moreover, if the therapist is unaware of autistic characteristics, they are unlikely to give credit to the client for the incredible amount of work being done in order to build a set of 'rules' by which the therapist, and indeed the rest of the neurotypical world, operates.

In order to build their 'rules' of behaviour, people with AS need to be astute observers, and they are often able to suss out aspects of a therapist's character that even the therapist didn't know! Once they feel comfortable with the way the therapist works and with the context in which they are interacting with the therapist, however, they are often well able to establish a working relationship. It just may not look like it in the beginning because the therapist is faced with an unsmiling, 'stand-offish', quiet person with weird eyes.

Indeed, this apparent inability to 'fit in' with others, as evidenced by the isolated childhood, is one of the main reasons people get referred for therapy. People with AS are frequently told, or shown by the behaviour of others, that they are odd, do not fit in, have little to contribute and are out and out wrong in the things they do. Managing to cope in a society that has a thousand and one ways to tell a person they are different takes its toll on the individual. As one person with AS said, 'If you hear a thing over and over and over, you start to believe it, become it, live it.'

Despite their best attempts to join in, people with AS are more typically bullied or ridiculed. Self-esteem therefore takes a tremendous beating (Edmonds and Worton 2005, 2006a, 2006b). If they then come to therapy and again meet with a therapist who tells them they are not 'doing it' right, their self-esteem takes another hit. If the therapist is convinced that the person needs to be more 'in touch' with their emotions, for example, and the person with AS simply cannot do this, then they are lined up for yet another failure. Seeds of inadequacy have usually been well and truly planted, and via misdirected problem focused therapy, for some individuals, the negative seeds can be nurtured and helped to grow. This is, we think, the way so many people, both with and without AS, become 'revolving door' patients who are long-term users of mental health services.

Sharing

People with AS may not know what things a therapist would like to know about, and as such they are people who 'hide their light under a basket'. Vicky remembers sweating with the effort of engaging a mother and daughter, both with AS, in a conversation about anything interesting or good that had happened since the last appointment. They could think of nothing, despite Vicky's prompts, and Vicky was getting dangerously close to the point where complimenting them on the very satisfactory nature of their breathing was about the best that could be done. Almost imperceptibly, Mum turned to the daughter and said quietly, 'Well, I guess you did save those two little girls from drowning.' 'Yeah,' her daughter said, 'but surely Vicky doesn't want to know about *that.*' Not want to know?! *Not want to know*?! Are you kidding?! The *pope* should know about that! Metaphorically speaking, Vicky leapt up with such excitement she knocked over her chair, fell to her knees and thanked the therapy god for sending such a gift as a person who can save children from drowning in order to get her out of a tight therapy spot. The pair were stunned by Vicky's aggressively enthusiastic reaction; we think they were the ones to recommend therapist sedation on their feedback form. (They were not exaggerating either. Once the entire story was told, it was clear that the young woman did indeed drag two children from a river. Ho-hum indeed!)

For therapists, this means that quite a lot of successes (and apparently child-saving episodes) are likely to go unreported unless the therapist specifically goes looking for them and stays on the trail until she finds them. People with AS may not think to initiate a conversation about what they have done well, but they certainly can respond to such a conversation if the therapist initiates it. Sadly the reverse is true, and if the therapist focuses only on the problems, the person with AS will also do that to the exclusion of all the good stuff that is happening.

Social give-and-take

The pesky little difficulty of not knowing what to share can spill into other social situations too, and a therapist may find that a person looks ill at ease in a waiting-room because of a difficulty in sharing space with others. They may fail to hold doors open for people, or not think to offer the use of a pen when someone is looking for one, and so on. Vicky has been choking, in the kitchen, near the sink, with a young man with AS and never been offered a drink of water. Not that the man was rude, he simply didn't connect her potential death with his ability to get water. It's an easy mistake to make. These kinds of differences in thinking may not directly impact upon a therapy session, but can certainly influence the opinion of a worker, should they be observing the person outside a therapy room. It isn't that the person with AS is ignorant or unkind. It is simply that they didn't think they would have anything useful to contribute to somebody else. It didn't occur to them. We can see the headlines: 'Psychologist chokes to death; client says "oh".'

Along similar lines, people with AS are often mortified to find themselves alone with a person who is in some kind of distress. The nature of the distress can be incapacitating in itself if it is in the form of loud wailing or hysterical motor activity or profuse bleeding and dying, for example. People with AS often recognize that something is expected of them in these circumstances, but they just do not know what to do. Emotional or physical distress isn't something that is easily quantifiable by rules, therefore the person with AS is left a bit high and dry on the 'here's-what-to-do' front. Again, this is not likely to have a huge impact on a therapy session unless the therapist is prone to collapse or choking (see above), but the person can certainly be misjudged by the therapist or others as a 'cold', 'unfeeling' person when a more apt descriptor would be 'unskilled'. It isn't that the person with AS doesn't want to help, it is that they do not know what to do for the best. Once they learn what to do, they are usually happy to do it, but such knowledge doesn't come naturally.

Therapy and communication

Just the facts please

Keeping with the theme of relationships, people with AS are not usually good at starting, maintaining or ending social interactions in the traditionally accepted ways. The quality of their social overtures can be pretty basic. Sometimes there is no 'hello' or 'excuse me', there is just a launch into whatever question or topic is on their mind at that moment. It is likely that they didn't think about a greeting because they were focused on whatever they were thinking. Likewise, sometimes conversations end when the person gets up and walks away. Vicky has had quite a few therapeutic encounters that end when the person walks away, leaving her standing (or sitting) like a lemon in an empty room with her own funny eyes and fish-like lips. A neurotypical therapist may find this kind of behaviour unacceptably unsocial, and may again find the person to be ignorant or unkind. It is more as if conversation has a function for a person with AS, and that function is to exchange information. Saying 'hello', 'excuse me', or 'goodbye' doesn't really impart any information, therefore it can be skipped. When an AS person begins to see these social niceties as functional, they are more likely to do them.

Social chat, such as one might have at the beginning of a therapeutic session, can also be difficult for an AS person. It can be hard to spot the functional and practical usefulness of social chat about the weather or time of day or holiday season, so it is hard for an AS person to know what information they ought to be contributing. Should they say everything they know about the temperature, the forecast, the weather trends for this time of year, or should they just say, 'Yes, the weather is awful' – which the speaker already knows? From an autistic perspective, they might just as well say 'blah blah blah' and then get on with the required conversation of the therapy. It needs specifically pointing out that social conversation helps the therapist to get settled into the session, for example. And, a person with AS could possibly do with some feedback as to how successful they were at their social chat which made the therapist feel more comfortable. Once developed, this is a skill which will hold them in good stead as they go forth into the cold, cruel world. Sadly, rarely do therapists think to do such a thing. Indeed it would be unusual for a therapist to own their own need for social chat, which would probably make sense to a person with AS. Usually the client is put down as 'asocial' because they do not behave 'normally', despite the notion that 'normal' behaviour often does not make a lot of sense.

Starting from different places

People with AS also sometimes have difficulty remembering that what they know in their mind is not necessarily in the mind of other people. In therapy this means that stories sometimes start in the middle because the client assumes Vicky already knows the beginning. Also, topics can shift with whiplash speed during a session as one thought triggers another thought related only in the client's mind. At these times the ability of the therapist to seek and achieve clarity with the AS person is critical. Rather than making the assumption that the client has 'fragmented thoughts' or 'pressure of speech', Vicky will assume half of the responsibility because she is not able to turn mental corners as fast as the client, and she will let the person know that she is not following what they are saying. People with AS are remarkably patient with Vicky in this regard, and are happy to revert to words of one syllable in order to bring her along with their thinking.

A lovely side-effect of the chronic checking of mutual understanding within solution focused work is that people with AS can soon adopt the same idea and keep checking with Vicky to see if she understands what they are meaning. And no matter how often her mind grinds to a standstill and says she doesn't understand, they pretty much keep explaining it until she does understand or the sun sets on their efforts, whichever happens first. In the main, people with AS are very patient, funny and helpful with people who listen to them, and ask questions in a genuine attempt to understand.

Along with the occasional rapid changes of topic, people with AS are prone to sudden interruptions of others in order to say what has just come into their minds before they forget it. This can be quite dispiriting to therapists who are trying to get through a spiel about one thing or another, but are interrupted by the client with off-topic statements. Vicky has been in the middle of imparting some positively brilliant observations to people with AS, only to be blown away by these sudden and intense interruptions about the Irish football team's new home kit or some other kind of thing. It's humbling on a good day and irritating on others.

If interruptions get too disruptive, Vicky has been known to reach an agreement with the client that they can make note of the interruption in writing, but won't discuss it until they have finished with their present topic. Another thing which sometimes helps is to agree that only one person gets to talk at a time, and that there is a clear signal about whose turn it is at any time. People with AS generally appreciate these kinds of boundaries being made explicit, even though a neurotypical therapist may feel mean by doing so.

People with AS are not intending to be rude by interrupting. It is a part of how they are wired to think and act, and as such it is part of what they bring to therapy. It is not a symptom of an underlying awful thing, and it is the responsibility of the therapist, in conjunction with the client, to find ways to make use of their way of working.

And finally, with respect to interacting with others, people with AS quite often exhibit inappropriate facial expressions, odd gestures or other socially unusual responses when interacting with others. This often has to do with the amount of anxiety or stress the person is under, and it can cause no end of difficulties. For example, when being questioned by police, people with AS often start to giggle, smirk or laugh. Not being known for their jolly sense of humour when investigating a crime, the police take this as disrespect for their authority (along with the shifty eyes as a sign of guilt) and AS people find themselves in jail for the night.

This mismatch of faces and emotions can be less dramatic but still problematic in a therapy session when a person's face or body appears inconsistent with what is being discussed. Again the labels of 'resistant to treatment', 'lacking remorse', 'disrespectful' and others get bandied about. These assumptions get made, and not checked out with the person. We find that when they are checked out, the person often does not know what emotion their face is registering. Vicky has often said, 'You look a little angry since I've said that,' or something similar, to which the person has replied with genuine surprise. A conversation can then ensue which clarifies things for both people. It seems critical for the therapist to take responsibility for thoroughly checking out their impressions with the AS person, especially because we know the AS person is using language differently and understanding things differently than a non-AS therapist.

Again, we make the point about listening closely and believing what the AS person says when asked questions such as, 'You seem upset... Are you?' Vicky observed one of her clients looking into the distance and moving his lips (and she noticed some fierce activity from his eyebrows too) as though he were having quite a heated discussion with someone. He was doing this while she was writing something in the notebook, so it was 'free mental time' from his point of view; he was not concentrating on interaction with Vicky at the time. Vicky observed this for a while, then asked the man what he was doing. He looked at Vicky like he'd woken from sleep and said, 'Pardon?' to which Vicky repeated the question and added, 'You looked like you were talking to yourself.' He said 'No. I was just thinking.' Vicky further checked this out by adding, 'You were moving your lips like you were talking. Were you talking to yourself in your head?' And again he said 'No. I was really just thinking.' Vicky did not then write in her notes, 'Patient can be seen talking to himself', as some therapists might have done. If the man says he's thinking, then he's thinking. Vicky's next step might be to let him know people can see him thinking because he's moving his lips and his eyebrows look sufficiently agitated to fly off and start a life of their own. It may make people look at him strangely, and he might need to know why they are doing that.

I love to talk

Another characteristic of AS is not knowing what information is of interest to other people. As one person seen by Vicky put it, 'I am bored rigid by other people's small talk, but absolutely fascinated by my own!' Such a person is likely to go on rather a lot about things of interest to them, without noticing the effect this is having on the people around them. There is a noticeable lack of 'give-and-take' with the conversation as the person with AS may not build on what the other person is saying, but continues with their own topic of conversation. It is easy to see how this can render talking therapy pretty ineffective in a very short time.

However, while the person is talking about the things that really interest them, Vicky, as a solution focused therapist, is able to listen out for, and collect, basketsful of characteristics that may be used to help the person reach the goals they want. People show aptitudes for noticing details, for memory, for mental manipulation of information, good spatial skills, good observational skills, amazing concentration and lots of other things which can be put to good use later in the work.

The difficulty of not building on what another person says may fox a few therapists, and by now the reader will know it is incorrect to assume the client is ignorant or self-centred because of this way they have of talking only about their own interests. Vicky has found that when people with AS feel listened to, they are more likely to do some listening themselves. In some cases, it has been helpful to write the topic of discussion on a paper and to point to it when the conversation is in danger of veering off track. In the main, people with AS want the benefit of therapy, so they are happy to be redirected to a topic which is useful to them. It is harder to direct them back to a topic which is not so useful to them, such as relaxation when the idea of relaxing does not mean anything to them. This is yet another reason why a common understanding of clients' goals is critical in order for therapy to work. A person is not going to be easily redirected to a topic that is only of interest to the therapist or the author of the 'how-to-do-psychology' books.

My language is unique to me

Often people with AS use words in a literal way. Telling a person with AS 'My head's all over the place' can result in some quite disturbing images if it is taken literally. Most language is full of turns of phrase that are not meant to be taken literally. For example, in one meeting where a neurotypical person was needing to leave, she said, 'Right, I'm going to shoot myself,' meaning 'Right, I am ready to leave (shoot off) and am going to go now.' The person with AS looked alarmed and asked 'Don't do that! Was it something I said?' which confused the person needing to leave. Vicky was on hand to explain that the woman wasn't going to take her own life, she was just having to leave the meeting. For days afterward the person with AS reflected on what an odd use of language that was.

Therapy and associated social conversation is full of such metaphorical use of language. 'Take a seat' springs immediately to mind, to which an AS person might honestly answer, 'Take it where?' or 'Take which one?' It is the stuff of which comedies are made, but when you live it every day, it becomes rather cumbersome. And when neurotypical people, who are hell-bent on having non-purposeful social chat and doing illogical things, try to make you feel like you are the one with the disability, it can be downright annoying.

It isn't that people with autism do not understand metaphors, puns or turns of phrase, so much as they do not know the rules about when to use them. We find that people with AS have very clever plays on words, and that much fun can be had using puns, metaphors and similes, when it is clear that these are part of the rules of engagement.

Again, the practice of checking for a mutual understanding of what is being said is the critical aspect for therapy. A therapist would do well, however, to pay close attention to their own use of words when giving homework ideas or making suggestions. One would not want a person with AS to *always* stop and think before they speak because they may be in the middle of a very busy road when they next wish to speak. We can again see the headlines: 'Person with AS killed by bus; therapist says "Oh".'

People also have unique ways of using language to describe aspects of themselves or their lives. Sometimes people with AS make up words, and it is important that the therapist understands the meaning and importance of those words. One example of such a word (and we kid you not) is 'Narskwediphairdog' which was used by one highly intelligent man to express confusion or exasperation. Again, we believe it is easier for the therapist to learn and use the language of the client (though not perhaps to use this particular word) than to expect the client to learn and use the language of the therapist.

One woman, when asked how Vicky would know if therapy was working for her, replied, 'By my hair.' 'Hair?' Vicky said. 'Hair,' she confirmed. It transpired that when she wore her hair loose she was feeling pretty relaxed, whereas if her hair was tied back she was anxious, and if it was French-plaited close to her head she was best avoided. So the more frequently she wore her hair down, the better she would be feeling. Said like that, it makes sense doesn't it? And it was as good a measure of success as we needed.

Therapy and perceptual/sensory differences

Interests

People with AS often have a narrow range of interests or have preoccupations which they pursue to the exclusion of other things. These are the things they love to talk about, of course, and as such they provide a rich source of information about their strengths and skills. Also, this narrow range of interests has an important bearing on the goals that are set for the therapeutic work. Goals that are typical of psychological therapy are often to do with anger management, recognizing and managing emotions, relaxation, managing relationships or something similar. A person with AS may not see the relevance of any of those goals. Vicky can remember trying to get people to follow relaxation programmes before she began working in a solution focused way, because it was obvious that the client was anxious in social situations. In the main, AS people didn't follow the relaxation programme, which was a source of frustration to Vicky. Once in a solution focused frame of mind however, when goals were negotiated, it became blindingly obvious that a person who was interested, say, in making new friends wouldn't see the relevance of using a relaxation tape! Goals which are framed within the person's own interests, using the person's own language, are far more useful than those framed in the therapist's language.

Rituals and routines

People with AS are often helped by their predictable rituals and routines. In terms of therapy, it makes sense, then, that people with autism get the same therapist, at the same time, on the same day and at the same place. It can also be helpful if the therapy follows a pattern which becomes easily predictable to the client. This is especially important early on, it seems, when the relationship with the therapist is not yet established.

Pre-solution focused days, Vicky used to assume everyone wanted to be seen every week as a matter of routine, but when starting solution focused work, people were given an option. Vicky started to ask the question, 'Would you like another appointment?' and if yes, 'How long do you think we should wait before we meet again?' To her great surprise and relief, people did not want to come every week! They usually said between four and six weeks later! Imagine that! Vicky was able to see more people, less often, and the waiting list disappeared within six months. In this sense, people do not have to be governed by 'sameness' as one might think. If in control and feeling secure, people with AS can tolerate quite a few changes in many routines.

I see the parts, but where's the whole?

As part of the way the connections are made in their brain, people with AS may find they are more attuned to details than they are to seeing the bigger picture made by adding the details together. They see the metaphorical 'tree' with no idea they are in a forest. Sometimes this is evident by their attention to the parts of an object, such as the wheel of a car. We think this same process may be evident when a person is not able to recognize how small achievements combine to make an overall goal. For example, a person who wants to drive may not intuitively understand the need to a) stop buying CDs so that b) he can save money so that c) he can afford driving lessons so that d) he can take a test so that e) he can drive. Neurotypical people often make these associations quickly and easily, while an AS person is left wondering how on earth the first thing relates to the last thing.

Likewise, a person with AS may not see how their behaviour of a) slamming the door led to Mum's behaviour of b) shouting at the person which made them c) swear at their mum which made her d) cry. This scenario is common if the person was coming in the door thinking of one thing, such as what just happened at college, and they do not even realise they slammed the door, so they have no idea why Mum is shouting at them, nor how their behaviour is involved in the end result of Mum crying. They would, understandably from their perspective, say that Mum was 'getting at' them and that she cries for no reason. Many times, though not all of course, we think this is why people with AS appear to blame other people for things that go wrong, even when they have done something to cause things to go wrong themselves. In their mind the sequence of events has not been put together.

My toes keep tappin'

Some people with AS move in order to keep their concentration. These people are 'fiddlers'. They will click pens, jiggle their feet, wiggle in their chairs (for goodness' sake think twice before seating them on a swivel chair with wheels), stand up, walk around, pick things up, and generally keep moving. Some therapists might see this as a lack of attention or not taking their problems seriously. They may feel that the person isn't respecting them enough to sit still and pay attention. More often, with AS it is the case that if the person sits still, they will fall asleep. Seriously. Moving helps them keep focused, aids memory, keeps their brain in processing mode and prevents a general system collapse. It is worth asking, and coming to a common understanding as to what movements will and will not interfere with the work. It is reasonable for the therapist and client to set some limits, and if done within the remit of collaborative working, most people with AS are happy to work within reasonable boundaries.

It may also be the case that the person with AS needs frequent breaks in order to move or twirl or flap or whatever it is they do to relax their mind. Again, this is an arrangement best made by negotiation. If a therapist asks a person with AS how long they can sit before they need to move about, the person with AS is quite likely to be able to tell them. If the therapist listens to them, then the movements need not mean that the person is 'unable to benefit from therapy', as might be assumed otherwise.

The bells...the bells...

People with AS often have sensory sensitivities (try saying that three times fast). Environments with bright or flickering lights, for example, can be very distracting to a person with autism. These lights may seem perfectly ordinary to a neurotypical person but can interrupt the ability of an AS person to process information. Likewise an environment which is noisy with chronic low-level noises, such as humming computers, or with sudden loud noises, such as car horns or slamming doors, can be brain-jarring for people with AS. Uninvited or surprise touch can be aversive, as can certain smells, or the movement of clock hands or computer screensavers. Offices may feel hot or cold to an AS person yet be comfortable for the neurotypical therapist. It is impossible to make an ordinary office free of all distractions, of course, and what bothers one person may not bother another. We mention these because a therapist who is aware of the distracting potential of sensory stimuli may be better able to have a conversation about how to minimize the distractions for an AS person.

Vicky has found more success in seeing people with AS in their own homes than in having them come to an office. Occasionally, an office visit is just the thing, but more often people feel much more comfortable in their own homes. Seeing where people live also gives a therapist even more information about the things that are important to that person, things that the person can do well, and clues about what the person does with their time between therapy sessions. Usually in their own homes, people have already dealt with sensory issues and they are able to concentrate on the tasks at hand, rather than scanning the new environment as they would do in an office.

Summary

- People with AS are not disabled by their autism, but by being in the company of inflexible, intolerant, uninformed people. This social model of disability fits nicely with the social constructionist philosophy of SFBT.
- Professionals diagnose autism by observing the presence or absence of behaviours which indicate difficulties with social skills, communication and behaviour.
- People with autism define autism by noting the internal states of information-processing problems, cognitive differences and sensory/perceptual differences.

- Autism is a difference in the way a person's brain is wired, which means that people with AS take in, store, retrieve and use information in different ways than their neurotypical counterparts.
- People with AS may have real mental health problems not because of AS but because they are in an inflexible environment, or for the same reasons non-AS people have these problems.
- Differences in social interaction may make the person with AS look disinterested, guilty, depressed and hard for a therapist to 'read'.
- Differences in communication may mean a lack of social chat, difficulties initiating and maintaining conversations with a therapist, interrupting the therapist, starting a story in the middle, interpreting language literally, using made-up words or talking at length about a special interest.
- Differences in sensory experiences and perception may be the reason why the typical office environment is uncomfortable, the person is unable to see how small steps combine to relate to an overall goal, or the person fidgets during therapy.

References

American Psychiatric Association (1994) *Diagnostic and Statistical Manual of Mental Disorders* (fourth edition) (DSM-IV). Washington, ED: American Psychiatric Association.

Beardon, L. (in press) 'Is autism a disorder?' Sheffield: The Autism Centre. Available at www.shu.ac.uk/theautismcentre (accessed 6 August 2007).

Bogdashina, O. (2006) *Theory of Mind and the Triad of Perspectives on Autism and Asperger Syndrome.* London: Jessica Kingsley Publishers.

Deudney, C. (2004) *Mental Health in People with Autism and Asperger Syndrome: A Guide for Health Professionals.* London: National Autistic Society.

Edmonds, G. and Worton, D. (2005) *The Asperger Love Guide.* London: Sage Publications/Paul Chapman Publishing.

Edmonds, G. and Worton, D. (2006a) *The Asperger Social Guide.* London: Sage Publications/Paul Chapman Publishing.

Edmonds, G. and Worton, D. (2006b) *The Asperger Personal Guide.* London: Sage Publications/Paul Chapman Publishing.

Ghaziuddin, M. (2005) *Mental Health Aspects of Autism and Asperger Syndrome.* London: Jessica Kingsley Publishers.

Gillberg, I. and Gillberg, C. (1989) 'Asperger syndrome: some epidemiological considerations.' *Journal of Child Psychology and Psychiatry 33*, 813–842.

Grandin, T. (1996) *Thinking in Pictures: and Other Reports from My Life with Autism.* New York: Vintage Books.

Kadesjo, B., Gillberg, C. and Hagberg, B. (1999) 'Brief report: autism and Asperger syndrome: a total population study.' *Journal of Autism and Developmental Disorders 29*, 4, 327–331.

Malloy, H. and Vasil, L. (2002) 'The social construction of Asperger Syndrome: The pathologising of difference?' *Disability and Society 17*, 6, 659–669.

National Autistic Society (2001) *Ignored or Ineligible?* London: The National Autistic Society.

National Institute for Clinical Excellence (2007) 'NICE Compilation Issue 10: Mental Health'. Available at www.nice.org.uk (accessed 6 August 2007).

Williams, D. (1996) *Autism: An Inside-Out Approach. An Innovative Look at the Mechanics of Autism and its Developmental Cousins.* London: Jessica Kingsley Publishers.

Wing, L. (1992) *The Triad of Impairments of Social Interaction: An Aid to Diagnosis.* London: National Autistic Society.

Wolfensburger, W. (2000) 'A brief overview of social role valorization.' *Mental Retardation 38*, 2, 105–123.

World Health Organisation (WHO) (1990) *International Statistical Classification of Diseases and Related Health Problems* (tenth edition) (ICD-10). Geneva: World Health Organisation.

Recommended reading

Attwood, T. (2006) *The Complete Guide to Asperger's Syndrome.* London: Jessica Kingsley Publishers.

Bogdashina, O. (2006) *Theory of Mind and the Triad of Perspectives on Autism and Asperger Syndrome.* London: Jessica Kingsley Publishers.

Department of Health (2006) 'Better services for people with an autistic spectrum disorder: A note clarifying current Government policy and describing good practice.' Available at www.dh.gov.uk/Publicationsandstatistics (accessed 6 August 2007).

Deudney, C. (2004) *Mental Health in People with Autism and Asperger Syndrome: A Guide for Health Professionals.* London: National Autistic Society.

Edmonds, G. and Worton, D. (2005) *The Asperger Love Guide.* London: Sage Publications/Paul Chapman Publishing.

Edmonds, G. and Worton, D. (2006a) *The Asperger Social Guide.* London: Sage Publications/Paul Chapman Publishing.

Edmonds, G. and Worton, D. (2006b) *The Asperger Personal Guide.* London: Sage Publications/Paul Chapman Publishing.

Chapter Four

Putting it all Together

The work of the Missing Link Support Services Ltd

We thought it might be useful, by way of giving even more detail about AS and SFBT (and to repeat our key points yet again!), to describe some of the solution focused work that has been done by Vicky at the Missing Link Support Services Ltd (MLSS), during one calendar year. In the section that follows Vicky describes some of the characteristics she has come across when working with people who have AS. These descriptions of practice are generalizations, and are not meant as rigorously collected research data. (Give us time to become rigorous with our data, we are only a young company!)

Fifty-six individuals between the ages of 18 and 65 with ASD were referred to the service; 66 per cent of these were male and 33 per cent were female. Under half of these people (25 or 44%) were referred for an assessment and diagnosis of ASD, whilst others were referred for depression, anxiety or relationship difficulties. The majority of individuals were in their twenties and thirties. Six men (10%) and one woman were known offenders. Referrals mainly came from someone else, so some people did not feel that they actually had a problem to be solved, or felt that the problem belonged to someone else. Still others felt that the problem was not solvable at all, or were eager to get Vicky to solve the problem for them. They clearly didn't know at that stage that Vicky really, really has an empty head and couldn't solve a problem for them even if she were required to!

Families were involved in just over half of the cases (53%). For the men, the number of sessions ranged between one and 21, with 32 (86%) of the men having between one and five visits. For the women, the number of sessions also ranged between one and 21, with the majority of women (13, or 68%) having between one and five sessions. The average number of sessions was three for men and six for women.

All but two of the men and two of the women stopped seeing Vicky on a professional bases, but seven men and two women attend the Tuesday Evening Social Club and see her informally there. Reasons for closure included assessment or therapeutic goals being reached for 33 (59%) of individuals and money running out for 16 (29%) individuals; two people moved away and one decided solution focused work was not for her. Four individuals are, as said above, still attending for sessions.

The first meetings generally went one of two ways; either the person was a great superficial talker (that is, knew social phrases and polite social body language) or they were quiet, withdrawn, perhaps suspicious-looking because of those funny ol' eyes. There often was little or no eye contact, although on occasion there was persistent staring at Vicky or another fixed point.

On a minority of occasions there was lots of movement, as in wiggling, tapping or crossing and recrossing legs, or even some rocking. Vicky usually opted not to worry about this, though later when rapport was established Vicky asked the client if she ought to be concerned about this movement as a sign of high anxiety or something else. The person with AS reliably said whether or not it was normal for them but always suggested that Vicky should not worry about it. The important thing was for Vicky to *believe* whatever they said about this, even if page 154 of the therapist textbook says this type of movement is characteristic of an anxiety disorder, obsessive-compulsive disorder, or some other diagnosable thing. Also, Vicky watched how the course of the conversation affected this movement, so as to learn what might increase or decrease it, in case the person later voiced a wish to do this. A therapist would be wrong to make the assumption that the person wants to stop these movements, without actually asking if this is the case.

Pre-session change seemed mainly to be a surprise question, and more often than not was met with a negative answer, 'Nothing's been better' – though later in the conversation there often were signs that some things had improved even before therapy began. This is not terribly different from the beginning of non-autistic first sessions.

Non-problem talk was often where the person with AS relaxed visibly, started making good eye contact, breathing rhythmically, and smiling. The movements, if present, might continue even if the person was content. Topics which people favoured over the year included trains, toilets, computers, cricket statistics, football, movies, music, specific pop bands, the law, medical conditions, and animals, though there is always room for interest in even more topics.

As mentioned earlier, encouraging people to talk about non-problem-oriented things may be one way for therapists or workers to learn to really listen to, and believe, what people are saying. This is the same for people with or without autism. When given space to ramble on, non-problem talk helped put people in a positive, energized frame of mind and, as mentioned earlier, provided a goldmine for Vicky to notice and name competencies. In addition, an intensive interest, which is usually something that makes the client feel 'odd' in the neurotypical world, was restructured through non-problem talk as something interesting and a vehicle for showing off all that was good about themselves. People say this felt good.

Without exception, the people seen by Vicky at MLSS over the past year were clever, creative, of strong will, and survivors of difficult situations. As we have said before, Vicky never failed, when listening to people with AS, to find copious amounts of strength, humour, coping skills and strategies which have helped to get the person through the almost inevitable history of bullying, abuse, disjointed learning opportunities and solitary life. It was at this stage that these attributes flowed from the person and were readily available for Vicky to collect.

Some people with AS, just like people without AS, told fantasy stories about themselves and their abilities. This is one way some people cope with difficult realities, but following SF principles it does not have to be 'uncovered' or labelled by the therapist.

Non-problem talk also helped to establish a good working relationship based upon the recognition of mutual expertise. As the reader will now know, underpinning SFBT is the belief that the worker and the client are equal in their expertise and in their ability to contribute to a workable way forward for the client. Vicky worked hard during the year to avoid holding most of the power and knowledge as the expert 'fixer' of the client, even when the client or their carers insisted on asking her for her expert opinion. Keeping attuned to the balance of power helped Vicky to follow the client's lead wherever possible.

It was noticeable that Vicky avoided what sometimes happened in her problem focused practice when she was working on one goal (say getting the client to relax) and the client was working on a different goal (say making more friends). When this happened it was perfectly reasonable that the client did not do the relaxation homework, because they couldn't see how relaxation would lead to making friends. In other situations this might lead the client to be labelled resistant or unable to benefit from therapy, when all along the problem was that commonly understood goals were not established. If the therapist is working with the client as an expert, and they are discussing and agreeing goals, this is not likely to happen. In the main, ideas for doing something different between sessions were taken up by the clients.

Moving the conversation along to developing a common understanding of what the person wanted in the future sometimes had to be done concretely. One example of this was, ‘I have enjoyed hearing about your interest in trains, and we have learned a lot about your skills. I need to talk with you about something different now. Can we move on to talk about something other than trains?’ This might have been necessary because the person had cognitively not been able to pick up subtle cues that Vicky wanted to move the conversation along. When asked clearly about moving to a different topic, people with AS tended to say ‘OK’ and resume their listening frame of mind rather than their talking frame of mind.

The Miracle Question was rarely helpful in its original form. On the few occasions Vicky asked it, people said it didn’t make sense, and in keeping with solution focused principles Vicky believed them and found a more concrete way to ask about preferred futures. Pretending that the problems have gone away is a different way of talking for people with AS and they may have genuine difficulties thinking about a future that is different from the ‘here and now’. A difficulty with ‘pretending’ may also interfere with a full exploration of this kind of question, as may being unable to see the logic in pretending things are different than they really are. Vicky found that making the question more concrete, and giving carefully considered multiple choice options, sometimes helped. For example, for a few people listing what they did on a typical day (or yesterday if they needed to be even more concrete) was pretty easy when asked specific questions such as, ‘What time did you get up? How did you decide what to wear? What did you do after you got dressed?’ and so on. We then went back to those points and Vicky asked, ‘If the problem that brought you here today went away, would you get up at a different time?’ to seek out what exactly would be different if the problems were solved. An advantage that an AS person may have over a neurotypical person in this regard is the patience to stick with this detailed kind of questioning!

Sometimes Vicky worried that the goals the person wanted to achieve were not possible, or were based in a client’s fantasy rather than reality. By asking genuine questions of the person, it became clear whether or not the nature of their aim was based in fantasy or in a reality shared with their carers. It occasionally felt a tricky situation where Vicky had to make a conscious effort to stay with the client’s reality despite evidence that carer reality was different.

Usually it paid off to stay with the client's frame of reference while working separately with the carers in their different frame of reference.

Probably about half of the time, the person with AS found preferred future questions really difficult and Vicky put her own view forward of how she would know when therapy is finished. This is OK in some instances because it is not good to proceed with therapy when neither of the parties has any idea what they are trying to do together. However, an even better option would be to use information already gained from the person during the session in order to make some likely guesses as to what will be the case when the problems have gone away. For example, 'We've discovered that you really like routine, so we might make a guess that if we have worked really well in therapy, one thing that will be different is that you will feel you have more of a routine to your day. Do you think that might be right?' Then Vicky kept checking back that this goal still made sense to the person as sessions progressed.

About three-quarters of the time the goals of the AS clients did not match with the goals of the carers or with social control services such as probation. There was sometimes a temptation to panic about this, but in reality it is not a problem unless the different goals are mutually exclusive, which actually seems to happen rather rarely. On the few occasions when it has happened Vicky was able to show the conflict clearly to the person and thereafter work around it.

In common with many people who do not have AS, goals of the clients were sometimes simply 'to get my mum/dad/social worker off my back'. This comes across as a different goal than Mum's goal of 'getting my son to be quieter in the house'. In the distant past, Vicky remembered a section of the professional textbook devoted to the client needing to admit to their problems, then agree to work on alternative behaviour, but in solution focused work she and the client were excused from acting upon such advice and were able to work with the goal set by the client. When the goal of 'to get my mum off my back' is implemented in reality, it is often simply another way of saying 'to do what my mum wants'.

Coping and exception questions followed the same concrete kind of basis by coming from something Vicky heard the person say while they were talking about themselves. This anchor in a concept the person has already grasped may have made it easier for them to process. Thus careful listening for any tiny hints of coping or exceptions to the problem needs to begin as soon as the person enters the therapy room.

Because people with AS may struggle to recognize the connection between discrete pieces of information, Vicky sometimes needed to make connections between what the client has said, what she has observed, and the statement they are now making. For example, 'You said you only came to see me because your mother wanted you to. You have also talked about how you remember your mother's birthday every year. Those two things suggest to me that you are a very caring person towards your mother. Do you think that is true?' whereas with neurotypical clients the therapist could more confidently assume these connections were being made without pointing them out.

This difficulty joining discrete bits of information together also needed to be addressed when deciding upon future action. Vicky needed to say something like, 'Because you said you wanted to make new friends, and we decided that people liked someone who turned up on time, I was wondering whether or not you might practise using an alarm clock to get up in the morning?' Otherwise the suggestion of a clock may not be understood within the context of making new friends.

Vicky found that scaling was most often a very helpful thing for people with AS. It suited their logical and concrete thinking patterns, and helped Vicky feel more confident with her understanding of where the person was at, and where they would like to be. Sometimes people struggled with the concepts of 'more than' or 'better than' but this was exceptional among people with AS. A rule of thumb for Vicky in her practice became 'When in doubt, or at a loss for what to do next, scale something'. It has not let her down in over six years of solution focused work!

Typical psychological sessions are about 50 minutes in length and take place in the therapist's office. Vicky's work varied in length and most often took place within the client's home. The length was determined to some extent by the client. Attending to such a conversation is exhausting for many people with AS and short sessions were more effective than longer ones when attention was short. On the other hand, there were almost always carers involved, and they required time to be heard too. In these instances it was easy to have a two-hour session, though most often the person with AS did not wish to attend for the full two hours.

Seeing people in their own environment paid dividends because often it decreased anxiety and increased the sense of equality in the work. Vicky came onto the home territory of the person rather than the person travelling to unfamiliar surroundings. Seeing the home of the person also gave Vicky more scope for noticing and naming competencies such as keeping the house tidy, choice of decor, and so on. Vicky estimated that over half of the people she saw had pets, ranging from birds to larger dogs, and it was advantageous to be comfortable working with animals in the session. It was acceptable, usually, to ask that the animals go elsewhere, however, if Vicky or the client found them too distracting. (Birds in particular can make a hell of a racket!) Likewise with other noises in the home, such as the TV or radio being on, Vicky found people receptive to requests to turn them off, though they might not have thought to do this without a prompt from her. This is not any different to doing home visits for people without AS, of course.

In typical by-the-book solution focused work, there is a five-minute break where the therapist leaves the room to confer with observers (a luxury Vicky rarely has, being the only employee of the company!) or to gather thoughts about the final section of the session. In the main, Vicky didn't do this with people who had AS, so we are not equipped to comment on the usefulness of this aspect of SF work. One of the reasons (quite apart from her own disorganisation) why Vicky did not use this break is because of the urge to be transparent about every aspect of the session. Leaving the person alone may easily give rise to suspicions about what the therapist is up to, but more likely it will signal the end of therapy for the person with AS. It will then require a lot of energy for them to restart their 'therapy thinking' in order to be ready to receive the important feedback at the close of the session. It seems better intuitively for Vicky to do her thinking and summarizing and wondering about what to do next while the client is present and listening. In addition, when doing sessions in the person's own home, they wouldn't be right to be suspicious of a therapist who just nipped into the kitchen, uninvited, to gather their thoughts (and some of the better silverware...).

SFBT did not solve the referral problems for every person who was referred to Vicky, though in all cases where feedback was received a good relationship was noticed by the clients. Vicky feels strongly that the use of solution focused approaches was the main factor in the establishment of a good working relationship.

Getting back to Mike

As yet another example of putting solution focused work together with AS, consider the following example with Mike. This is about the third session together and he has spent most of those sessions talking about how badly treated he is by his family and friends. He has a family member, Chris, who has tried to keep in touch by phone and by visiting. Mike sometimes asks Chris to do favours for him, like take him shopping in the car or help him fix his computer, and Chris is happy to do these things.

Mike gives Chris bottles of wine or chocolates in order to say thank you, but Chris responds by saying, 'Oh, you shouldn't have gone to this trouble, Mike,' which makes Mike feel like he has done the wrong thing by trying to be nice.

Chris often asks Mike why he doesn't get out more, dress in newer clothes, buy more fish to eat, and clean his flat. Mike perceives these worries as digs at him. He thinks that Chris believes him unable to look after himself. Chris is genuinely concerned about Mike and truly unaware that the way he phrases things has a negative impact on Mike. Mike feels driven to aggressive behaviour which upsets Chris, and both end up saying very hurtful things. Chris ends up saying exactly what Mike doesn't want to hear. When upset, Chris does indeed say that Mike will never be able to look after himself and that no other member of the family will stand by him like Chris has.

In the following exchange, Mike and Vicky are talking about a joint visit they had with Chris when Mike and Chris ended up hitting each other. Both feel very bad about this but feel it is an inevitable part of their relationship that they will be angry with each other.

M: Yeah…the last time when he was here…when I…when I completely lost it…went completely over the edge you know…

V: Yeah…yeah, I know.

M: He was really being hard on me, he was absolutely cutting me to ribbons…he was really destroying me. I felt agonizing…really intense agonizing pain in my mind. He brought up all the pain that I'd been through… I remembered it… I remembered sitting in the car and…going on these long distances…and the pain…and all the long days of suffering…and blaming it all on to me…and even times when he wasn't there…and blaming everything on to me and other people.

He says, 'Oh I love you and you're my favourite member of the family,' and all this kind of tosh… Well, he has a very funny way of showing it…you know…it's like…

V: Because he brings you your shopping?… He rescues you at two in the morning if you are lost… That's how he shows he loves you… That's not weird is it? That's exactly what you would do if you loved someone, isn't it?

M: Yeah but it's like…it's the way he always seems to blame me for everything and that's the problem…like…why does he always come down like a ton of bricks…?

V: Yeah. Well. I only heard him giving his point of view, which was different to your point of view. It doesn't make either one of you right...just different. It must have been hard for you, otherwise you wouldn't have behaved like you did...so it must've been really hard for you. I didn't realise that that was the case...I didn't hear him giving you all the blame.

Vicky is not simply agreeing with Mike here but she is identifying her confusion about Mike and Chris's relationship. Chris seems to genuinely care for Mike and genuinely not recognize the part he plays in Mike's behaviour. When Mike tells him he is hurting him, Chris says 'No, I'm not', or 'Don't be so stupid'. Both points of view are correct; Chris does love Mike *and* he does not listen in a way Mike recognizes. Vicky is not suggesting what Mike says is wrong, but is admitting her inability to understand his point of view entirely.

M: All you...all you seem to get is the words. You hear the words. You didn't feel the pain... You didn't get...

V: I didn't, no... I wouldn't, would I, because I'm not emotionally involved. You're absolutely right, I only get the words and I'm thinking, well, that doesn't sound too bad...

M: Cos I'm getting the memories back... I'm going through all what I've been through. I mean, you're only hearing the words aren't ya?

V: Yes...yes exactly. That's a very good way to put that. And in those words only, things didn't seem too unreasonable but in the reliving it must've felt awful...

This is a lovely distinction and quite a good explanation for Vicky's confusion. Mike says the reason she doesn't understand is because she is only getting half the message he is. What he says is absolutely correct.

Jumping to later on in the session:

V: You're conscious of the fact that you keep causing stress did you say?

M: Aye...well...y'know...I'm conscious of the fact that I'm... um...you know...causing...well...I dunno...in somebody else's eyes I'm causing...I dunno...mischief or something...

V: Yet in your eyes, you're just standing up for yourself?

M: I'm just standing up for myself. I'm going 'What? What am I doing wrong here?' I think to myself. It's like…it's like a what was it? … (*unintelligible*)…but at the end of the day it's like…a…I say to him…look now…you're doing my flippin' head in…you're causing me grief…you're causing me aggro…you've done all this…you know…I've had all these hurts and things to me.

And he comes back with 'Well you've hurt me' and the only thing, the only way I can think of is that I'm trying to stick up for myself. Well if someone is being awful to ya you're gonna say that aren't ya? You're gonna say, 'Oh you've done all these mean things to me.' You're not gonna say, 'Oh thanks…you've been nice to me' are ya? I mean what are you supposed to say? How you supposed to stick up for yourself?

Oh…it just seems to give me extra suffering you know… I…I can't win.

It seems clear that there are a number of things which Mike does not understand. It is tempting to simply tell him how the world works. Tell him that he is taking what Chris says too literally, and that much of what Chris says are simple 'turns of phrase', such as when he says, 'Oh Mike, you shouldn't have bought me this wine'. It is hard to explain why Chris says this when he doesn't actually mean it literally. Likewise it is hard to explain to Chris why him saying this causes such deep distress for Mike.

M: Yeah well, at the end of the day if he's not appreciating that…what I'm doing, what I'm thinking is that, um, you know, like a gesture… That means he's not appreciating what I'm doing. Again it's like you can't win…

V: Yeah…I'd expect Chris to answer, if I said, 'How could Mike say "thank you" to you…I guess Chris'd say something like 'By not getting angry with me.' In your language he would be saying 'By not sticking up for himself', which…

M: Ahh (*chuckles*) by not sticking up for myself.

V: Which of course is not acceptable, it's not really…

M: Well then I can't win… I either bottle it up – stick up for myself…can't win…it's very very very suffocating…very stifling…you just get to the point where you can't handle this any more, all these dark thoughts come into your mind and you think

> the whole world is against you and you live in a very stressful life, and it's very hard because with people like that it's very agonizing and I sit here just dwelling on it and it gives me agonizing pain, it does.

Poor ol' Mike. He says it is helpful for him to talk about this stuff every time Vicky visits because he gets it all off his chest. He is working on noticing what he does differently after having got everything off his chest because this is something he has never paid attention to before, and it is important to notice and name what happens that's better so that he can start to try to do more of those things. We hope it is evident that Vicky is making an effort to listen closely to what Mike says and to believe that he knows what he is talking about, even when it doesn't make complete sense to her. Vicky's ears sometimes smoke and droop after a good day of hard listening such as this.

Service-oriented support

Because solution focused work relies so much on working with whatever is presented, and relies so much on the worker listening carefully and skilfully to whatever the person says, using the approach for people with AS requires no specific adaptations. It is one case, however, when a worker who is experienced in understanding the information-processing difficulties of a person with AS will probably do better than one who is completely unfamiliar with AS.

In this respect, specialist support services for people with AS are quite important. Unfortunately it is more typical around AS that person centred individually oriented solutions often lose out to service or condition centred solutions. The irony being, of course, that it is the individual differences of the person that earn them the label of AS, so it logically follows that the required support cannot be oriented for the benefit of the service over the benefit of the individual.

The report from the Department of Health (2006) 'Better services for people with an autistic spectrum disorder: A note clarifying current Government policy and describing good practice', recommends person centred and solution focused approaches as being something that should not be a rarity for a lucky chosen few, but should be available for all people with ASD. For its use of SF approaches with people who have ASD, MLSS is cited as a 'provider of choice' in the report (pp.39–40).

Summary

We think that SFBT and AS make an excellent match, and preliminary results from clients of MLSS support this belief. Solution focused work allows the therapist to bend around the strengths, needs and goals of the client in a way that makes therapy accessible to people who have the information-processing, cognitive, sensory and perceptual difficulties of autism.

References

Department of Health (2006) 'Better services for people with an autistic spectrum disorder: A note clarifying current Government policy and describing good practice.' Available at www.dh.gov.uk/Publicationsandstatistics (accessed 6 August 2007).

Chapter Five

Solution Focused Approaches in Everyday Life

Introduction

Therapy is not the only type of support required by people who have autism. Indeed, therapy is but one tiny fraction of a person's life, leaving the bulk of the support to fall in other areas. In this chapter, we begin a discussion about how the philosophies and techniques of solution focused therapy might be brought to bear on other areas of life, including employment, education and relationships. There is evidence, both in literature (Department of Health 2006; Edmonds and Worton 2005, 2006a, 2006b; Hesmondhalgh and Jackson 2006; Mayer 2001; Powell 2002) and in our own experiences that these three areas often provide sticking points for people with AS, and it may be that some aspects of solution focused work can help in these different settings.

Employment

Happy employment situations for people who have AS are a rare and beautiful thing. It is a sad state of affairs that people who are so talented, intelligent, diligent and thorough are not given a chance to show what exceptionally dedicated employees they can be. In the main, it seems that the reason employment is so difficult to secure and maintain for people with AS is because fellow workers automatically assume everyone is just like they are. Neurotypical workers, as a herd, are not very tolerant of different-ness, nor are they very flexible in their thinking. For example, people with AS may stare at someone while they are trying to process information about what that neurotypical person is doing. The 'normal' person automatically assumes that the person doing the staring has threatening intentions towards them, which is probably the farthest thing from the AS person's mind. A simple, single snowflake of an incident like this can quickly become a blizzard where no one can see the misunderstandings that are building up to an inevitable avalanche. It is such a shame, and an avoidable one at that. We know of people with AS who occupy a variety of positions, including general practitioner, detective inspector, psychologist, computer programmer, grants officer, teacher, taxi driver, administrative assistant, gardener and nursery nurse, to name just a few. There are a few we know who are self-employed. In the main, people who have jobs tolerate the needs of their neurotypical co-workers but it is not usually a completely happy situation. Sadly, we know even more people with AS who have moved from job to job because of bullying, misunderstandings about rules, differences of opinion and so on, or who have been unable to get employment at all.

Rarely do employers seek outside help in order to make reasonable adjustments to job descriptions in order to accommodate the differences of people with AS. When employers do seek our advice, we find that a number of very simple, low-cost adjustments can be made, so that the employer gets to keep an excellent employee and the employee gets to keep a regular source of income without losing their sanity in the process. One or two small changes in the way information is presented to an AS employee can make a very big difference.

So how might solution focused approaches be useful when supporting someone in employment? An obvious application would be for the support worker or manager to listen closely to, and believe, what the AS employee says about their work. If the employee says they enjoy their work, but the manager's observation is that they never ever smile or engage in conversation with anyone, there will be a temptation for the manager to discount what the employee says and assume that the person really does not like their employment. Whereas if the manager was visited by the solution-focus fairy overnight, they would have an exchange something like this:

Boss: So, Mike, I notice you don't really talk much to the people here. How are you enjoying your first week at work?

Mike: It's fine.

B: Are you getting along with people OK?

M: Yes.

B: How do you know if people like you?

M: (*After several 'dunno's' no doubt*) If they talk to me or smile at me.

B: Ahh...and do people here talk to you or smile at you?

The boss might continue with more solution focused, detail-oriented questions such as 'How will you know if you are doing a good job?' or 'How do you usually cope with not understanding something?' and then listening to and remembering the answers, so that the person gets the kind of feedback on their behaviour or their performance that will make a difference to them. Too often support workers or managers give feedback to AS employees in a way which ought to make sense, but is simply meaningless to the person with autism. The employee may *not* tell their boss that they don't understand something, perhaps because they have been conditioned to think that not understanding is their fault, and so a spiral of low self-esteem begins. Also, most people with AS do not wish to call attention to themselves, so they are not likely to admit a lack of understanding when everyone else seems to know what they are doing.

We cannot emphasize enough the importance of being genuinely interested in the answers to questions, and of believing what the person says. People with AS will know things about themselves that the rest of us will never understand, but in the main they are very patient with their explanations when they feel the listener is genuinely interested in understanding. And listening to the employee allows solutions to difficulties to be developed without the support worker or boss needing to know how to solve every problem. How good is that?!! No longer do 'those in charge' have to know the answer to every problem that arises. What they do have to know how to do is to listen, believe, and try to understand their employees.

Likewise, in terms of teaching an AS employee the requirements of the job, this can be made pretty easy by asking the employee how they learn best. Obviously then a worker or manager would want to co-construct a way for the person to learn about the jobs they need to do. It may be that the person learns best when in a quiet environment, but can then transfer them to a noisy one once they have mastered the skills. It may be that they remember things better if they both see and hear the instructions, though some people may remember well just by hearing instructions. Some individuals may learn best with hand-over-hand instruction initially, because they remember and learn best by doing the task. Frequently, people with AS do well with cues such as pictures that can be put up when there is a job to do, and taken down when the job is done. This helps them recognize and plan what is yet to do, as well as appreciate the amount they have already done.

AS employees may need their managers to give them a context and logical reasons for what they are doing. Putting information into a context is much like the person having a box in their head into which they store information about the job. If the context is 'clean toilets = happy manager', then a list of what makes 'clean toilets' can be stored in the 'clean toilets' mental box in the AS employee's head, or even on a visual list in the toilet area or some other handy place. Without this context, the employee may just hear their job duties as unconnected words to which they are unable to attach the overall meaning.

Luckily for workers and managers everywhere, people with AS can usually tell someone exactly how they learn things best. If they cannot, the manager can have a discussion with them about something they have already learned and ask them to recall how they learned to do it. The worker can also keep checking back with the employee to see if the method of instruction is working OK, or if changes need to be made.

We have come across people who fail to maintain their employment because their performance over all the tasks of their job is uneven. It is often the case that an AS employee will excel at one aspect of the job, such as data entry or policy writing, but really struggle with others, such as taking phone messages or recognizing when messages are urgent and warrant interrupting someone. Solutions to these uneven skills will probably be as individual as the employees and the businesses involved. One step in the right direction might be for both the manager and the employee to identify the detail of how they will know when the employee's performance is improving even one little bit higher on a scale in solution focused terms. That way the employee knows exactly, in measurable and observable terms, what they need to do in order for the boss to be pleased. It will be important for open dialogue with the employee to occur so that ineffective methods of improving the work are not continued.

A person with AS may not tell their support worker or their boss that a method of teaching is not working, as they often assume it is their fault and they keep trying harder and using up their energy to 'get it right'. It is usually more productive if the energies of the employee are directed into finding a better method of learning, remembering and executing a task.

It may be that creative solutions to the uneven performance are found through talking and listening as the employee tells about what things have worked in the past. Indeed, if the boss or worker identifies exactly how they will know when the job has been done satisfactorily, it may be that other means of getting the job done are found. For example, it might be that a piece of equipment can do the job, or it may be that tasks might be switched with other employees, so that the AS person does only tasks suited to their skills. It is worth remembering that effective solutions are not necessarily related to the definition of the problem.

Frequent feedback on the performance of the AS employee seems to be advisable, though how frequent would be determined by the realities of all involved parties. Feedback solution focused style would always include statements such as 'One thing I really like about your work here is…' or 'I noticed the other day that you talked to that customer really nicely'. It is easier then to follow this up with something like 'One thing that would make your work even better is…'. Remember that solution focused workers prefer the glass that is half full, so workers or bosses who are continually looking out for moments when the AS employee shines will reap more benefits than employers who only notice when things go wrong.

It might be helpful for workers or bosses to decide exactly what they will be seeing when they know that the employee is doing a good job. Readers will recognize this as identifying a preferred future, and as such the Miracle Question might be a good thing to try. For example, 'Imagine that when you go to sleep tonight, something wonderful happens to your AS employee. Because this wonderful thing happens overnight, you do not know it has happened until you see the employee the next day at work. What will you notice about the employee's work that will tell you something wonderful has happened to them and they are doing an even better job for you?' Perhaps the employee will smile? Perhaps the other workers will say complimentary things about the employee? Perhaps all the boss's messages will be given correctly? There are a number of possible things that would tell the boss that the AS employee's work was improving. Once these are identified, they can be discussed with the employee so that ways of making the boss's dreams come true can be developed.

Sometimes the little difference that makes a big difference is something like telling the AS employee it would make the boss feel great if they smiled and said hello when they come in to work. People with AS don't often know that their behaviour can affect others, so they simply may not have thought about this before.

Bosses and support workers can also use scales to keep track of where they think the training and work of the AS employee is up to. It would be applied exactly as it would in a therapy setting. For example, the support worker could rate their impressions of the employee after the first day, with ten being 'absolutely confident' and zero being 'absolutely not confident' that the AS person will get the hang of the job. Once the AS person has rated their own confidence level, they can think about the good things going on that give them that level of confidence. These are things the support worker wants to be sure keep happening with the employee. They can also decide what will have happened when their confidence improves just one little step. Identifying these things really does make it easier to notice when they do happen.

People with AS generally like boundaries put in place for them, so that they know what is expected of them. A good proportion of AS people also seem to struggle with taking directions or engaging in any meaningful way with people in superior positions to them. They often come into a job with a lifetime of experience in being bullied, made fun of, being different and feeling ineffective in many areas. They sometimes come across as resenting authority, though a worker ought not assume this simply from what the person says or how they say it. Remember that people with AS do not always understand the connection between the saying of words and the speed or tone in which the words are said. They also do not understand personal space sometimes, so they may stand too close, which would add to the feeling of threat to the worker. Simple, clear rules often work a treat. If the employee says it would be helpful, the reasoning behind the rule and the consequences of breaking the rule can be explained, though not everyone would want this depth of information. A question the worker and employee could discuss might be 'How will we know when we have the structure just right for you?' The person with AS may envision having a support worker with them for the rest of their lives, whereas the support worker may see their intervention as short-term. Unless the questions are asked and the discussions are open and equal, misunderstandings can fester.

Doing the tasks associated with the job may be the least of the employee's difficulties. There will be unstructured time during lunch and breaks when a person with AS is likely to find socializing difficult. Managers or support workers need to be mindful of this aspect of the job as well, and to keep an open dialogue with the employee about how he sees himself fitting in with the rest of the gang. It might be useful to use a scale to rate how supported or accepted he feels by his co-workers, being sure to agree the point on the scale that the AS employee feels is 'good enough'. AS employees may not want to be at a full ten in terms of support from other workers. A five or a seven might be good enough.

Education

Many of the same approaches would probably apply in the world of education. We work mainly with adults, so our focus is on higher education, but solution focused ideas have already been applied in school settings (e.g. Ajmal and Rees 2001). As with employment, the successful running of educational institutions requires that everyone follow the same basic structure. Classes have a beginning and an end which probably can't be varied too much to suit individuals. There is conduct which is acceptable at a college or during class, but this conduct is not often explicitly identified. People with AS struggle to know what behaviour is appropriate in different settings, so if it is possible to identify a code of conduct with the person, that may indeed be helpful. This code probably would need to include what to do in class if one has a question, what to do if one is confused, whether or not it is possible for someone to leave the class if they start feeling too anxious, and so on.

One of the common difficulties in higher education is the looseness of the structure. A student may have one class in the morning, free time, then one class later in the afternoon. A person with AS may struggle to fill free time in a safe or productive way. One of the aims of a support worker in this situation would probably be having a discussion with the person along the lines of 'How will we know if we get the amount of support just right for you?' and maybe 'How will we know if you are using your free time wisely?' We hardly need say it by now, but the critical aspect of this discussion is to listen to what the person has to say about these things.

Schools and colleges are full of a variety of people and there is ample opportunity for bullying to occur. People with AS probably have their own definition of bullying, so before talking about this kind of subject it would be helpful to reach a common understanding of what everyone means when they use the term 'bullying'. The worker could offer several scenarios to the AS student and they could discuss whether or not the student considers them bullying. This might also be a good way to begin learning how the student thinks situations of bullying might be best dealt with.

Scales could be used to assess confidence in handling bullying, and it would be good for the support worker to know what the student thinks needs to happen in order to increase their confidence one little step. It would also be good for the student to say what role the worker might play in handling a situation of bullying. Some people with AS would want a worker to intervene and some would be embarrassed for the bully to know a support worker was needed. Workers can also talk with the student about their own worries with regard to bullying. For example, if Vicky were a support worker, she would have to say to the student that if the bully is a big, angry person, she might feel a little frightened at the idea of direct action! If the student asks anything of the worker that makes the worker uncomfortable, an honest and equal discussion is called for.

How to support a person during a free period or during class time can be a delicate arrangement. Some students do not mind everyone knowing they have a support worker, and others would rather turn blue than admit to needing a support worker. Luckily, the worker can be equally successful with either student, so long as open and equal discussion has occurred about both what the student wants and what the worker needs to, or can, provide. People with AS are usually quite able and willing to negotiate on matters like these, so long as they are having expert-to-expert discussions on possible solutions. Workers need to feel free to talk to the person, perhaps after each class initially, in order to check out with the student whether or not they handled the situations in the best way. See? People with AS are there to help us workers every step of the way! We never have to make a decision alone, which is exactly how good support work should be done.

Relationships

Social relationships are at the heart of nearly everything a person wants to do. Even spending time alone may require some negotiation with another person. Many people with AS are lonely and would like to make friends but are unsure how to go about doing so. Many have histories of relationships gone wrong, but do not know exactly what happened to cause the breakdown. Some have developed ideas in their own mind about what happened, and it is important that these ideas are taken seriously, even when the worker doesn't understand quite where they came from. Not everyone *wants* to be 'normal' and be able to make small talk or have a lot of friends. In fact, what seems more common is that people with AS want to maintain their individuality sometimes but blend in with the crowd at other times. A standard question from Vicky when people say they want to make some friends is 'How many friends would be enough?' and 'How do you decide whether or not someone would make a good friend?' and 'How do you decide if you want to be one of the crowd or if you would rather assert your individuality?'

Solution focused approaches can provide a framework for support workers to unpick what it is the person with AS wants from relationships. Vicky worked with one man, for example, who said he wanted to meet women. In an uncharacteristic lapse of solution focused thinking, Vicky did not check her understanding of what he meant, and assumed he meant he wanted some women friends. Vicky started talking to him about the people who attend our Tuesday Evening Social Club and began describing, at his request, some of the women who attended there. After about five minutes of increasingly confusing conversation, during which the fellow asked questions about the physical characteristics of the women he might meet at the club, Vicky kicked back into SF mode and checked her understanding of what he really, *really* wanted. What he really wanted, as it turned out, was a girlfriend and what he really, *really* wanted was sexual intercourse. Ah. It was just as well that that got clarified before any introductory meetings were arranged. Rest assured that any subsequent discussions about meeting new friends involved a thorough and frank discussion about exactly what kind of friends were being talked about, as well as the precise nature of the shared activities he was planning to do.

People's lives take peculiar directions, and someone who has AS is no different from anyone else in this regard. Support workers need to believe, in their heart and right down to their shoes, that the AS folk they are supporting are doing their very best in any given situation. Lapses in judgement, concentration and motivation are to be expected both from the worker and from the person with AS. When the worker can acknowledge their own lack of experience, discomfort, or any other situation which might impact on the support they give, open dialogue can occur with the person who has AS.

We have sometimes heard about situations where the support worker's discomfort has meant that opportunities for the person with AS have been limited. A simple example would be Vicky going with a lovely, fun young woman to the zoo. The lovely, fun young woman wanted to go into the bat cave, and Vicky very much wanted to support her, but in the end it was either throw up with anxiety or run from the cave, and Vicky chose the latter. Fortunately a mutually respectful relationship had already been established between the pair and, once Vicky could breath normally again, she was subjected to much good-natured teasing from the person with AS. If that situation had happened in a parallel universe where an equal and respectful relationship had *not* been developed, Vicky might have been tempted to make up excuses for why the woman was behaving unreasonably by wanting to go into the freaky bat cave in the first place. Quickly and easily the person with AS could have had their confidence undermined because the 'person in power' had put the blame on them for being unreasonable. *Support worker: Know thyself and to thine own self be true* would be the moral of that little story. That, and Vicky hates bats almost as much as supermarkets.

It is so much easier to admit one's own shortcomings to a person with AS (or even a person without AS, come to that) when a respectful, honest relationship has been developed. This means, of course, that the person with AS gets to admit their own shortcomings too, without fear of penalty from the support worker. For example, the support worker might be gagging for a drink and suggest to the person that they go into a café for a coffee. The person with AS might say, though, that they do not want to go into the café because it is too crowded, or maybe for a reason they cannot even identify. In a respectful relationship, no one gets blamed for being a human being. By using solution focused approaches and working hard to establish a good working relationship, the support worker can help provide good 'on-the-job training', as it were, for the development of good social skills, which in turn will enhance relationships for the person with AS.

Solution focused approaches can be adapted to help someone with AS overcome difficulties in relationships, or even end relationships, if that is what the person wants to do. This relationship work can be tricky, of course, because the support worker also has a little role as 'the voice of reason' and as an agent of social control. If a person with AS is becoming agitated with other people, the support worker needs to feel confident about when to impose some structure to ensure the safety of everyone. Ideally the worker and the person with AS would have discussed the best course of action in the event that the person with AS lost control, and this discussion would have allowed the person to tell the worker how to identify when they are in danger of losing control. Workers can usually listen to and learn from the person with AS about when they are reaching their irrational state, because the person with AS usually knows themselves quite well. The person with AS may also have experience of past interventions at this stage which have worked well, and interventions which have not worked so well. We have found that, so long as they feel safe to do so, people with AS are remarkably candid about their occasional lack of self-control, as well as about approaches that do and don't work when they are in this state.

So a support worker needs to know how to recognize the moment when they need to step in and take direct action to keep people safe, and they need to know clearly what action to take, as well as how to take it. They need to know how to recognize if their intervention has worked, which may not be as straightforward as one might think. You, as the reader, will know by now that the key to knowing the answers to all these difficult issues is having an honest and respectful discussion with the person (and you may be jolly well sick of us repeating ourselves in this regard). We have found that people with AS are usually willing to think through a 'twenty questions' type of routine if they know that by doing so, they will help to ensure their own safety and help the support worker to feel more confident. This is a generous gift from the person with AS to the worker, because it means the worker can asked detailed questions such as:

> 'What will I see you do, or hear you say, if you are starting to get agitated and need me to step in?'

If the person doesn't know the answer to this, the worker might try:

> 'Can you remember the last time you needed someone to intervene for your safety or for that of others, and can you tell me what you were doing or saying, or even what your face was like when you were getting so upset?'

If the person cannot do this, perhaps:

> 'See that person on the TV? They look like they are about to lose control. Do you think that is what you look like when you need me to step in?'

Honestly, we are frequently surprised by the thoughtful comments people with AS are able to make when given these types of questions. Also (we could probably all recite these next questions together by now!) the support worker may ask:

> 'If I step in, how will I know that I have done the right thing? What will you say or do that will tell me I have handled the situation well?'

Again, we have been surprised by the variety of answers we get to this question. Some people will say that if the situation has been well managed, they will quickly walk away. Some people will say that they will calm down straight away, while others will say that they will pace or flap or do something else as they start to wind down. A worker could interpret a quick exit or some of these other behaviours as a sign that they had not handled the situation well, so it saves a lot of worry if this can be cleared up via a coherent discussion. Again, workers can keep asking questions and checking their understanding for as long as the person can keep coming up with answers.

Professional boundaries

We have found what we think is an unnecessary amount of damage done to people with AS in the name of 'professional boundaries'. Professionals have ethical guidance about using self-disclosure, about giving out personal information and about the dangers of getting 'too close' to their clients. Support workers are often called upon to make quick decisions about what information to share about themselves, or how to keep some information from clients who very much want to know about their personal lives. It seems unfair to ask clients to open up every aspect of their lives to us as staff yet give nothing personal back to them in return. We are asking them to trust us with their personal information, yet we do not trust them with our personal information.

On the other hand, staff are there to do a job for a client, and as such they are expected and paid to manage confidential information. Clients are not paid to manage confidential information about the staff, and we ought not to expect them to know how to do so. In support work, as in life, there are no easy answers. We do, however, think that workers need to address this issue because it is difficult, we think maybe even impossible, to establish an equal, respectful relationship without mutual disclosure of some personal information.

Indeed, the relationship with direct care staff is one of the most effective teaching tools available to support workers and people with AS. It is within this safe environment that people with AS are supposed to be able to practise socially appropriate behaviour, and this rich source of possibility will be severely curtailed if staff cannot respond in a give-and-take way.

One of the rules which we operate by, regarding self-disclosure, is that it always, yes *always*, is done thoughtfully and with the interests of the person with AS in mind. It is never acceptable for staff to unload their own private traumas and dramas onto people for their own personal satisfaction or gain. We are there to help people with AS, so the first rule of self-disclosure would be to ask, how is this helping the person? The second rule of self-disclosure, from our perspective, is, if it feels uncomfortable, tell the person that, along with why you are uncomfortable, and then get the client's views on whether or not they need to know. Most people with AS will be perfectly reasonable, if they understand about staff worries, and will not feel slighted if staff do not answer all of their questions.

What we think does not contribute to the equal and mutually respectful relationship is an automatic shut-down response from staff, such as 'I am not allowed to discuss that with you', or 'We are not here to talk about me', or 'I don't see how that information is relevant to your situation', or something similar. If staff talk to people with AS in that way, they can expect people with AS to talk to them in that way.

A final word about SF questions

In response to solution focused questions, the most common answer is 'I dunno'. The questions are unusual and require a person to think quite a lot before answering. Many people, with and without AS, do not have practice in thinking about how they do things right, or how they get bad situations to go away. We are more used to talking about the problems than about our magnificent coping skills for managing the problems. When first learning to use solution focused questions, workers get a little panicked when a client says 'I dunno', because it can be hard to know where to go from there. Giving the person a few seconds, or minutes even, to think about the questions is fine. A little silence is not harmful, even if it feels uncomfortable. Sometimes Vicky says, 'I dunno either. How do you think we could find out?' or 'Who do you think might know?' or sometimes Vicky will give some options. One thing to be careful of when giving options, though, is always to have one option be 'none of the above', because none of the offered options might fit.

Summary

- So, solution focused approaches are not just for Christmas. (Ha, only kidding.)
- Solution focused approaches are not just useful in the therapy room. They can provide a helpful framework for establishing a good working relationship with someone who has AS in a variety of settings.
- They can help both the person with AS and the worker recognize signs that they are doing the right things. They can help both of them to identify their own, and their joint, preferred futures. They can help both of them to identify what things are already working well, or what things worked well in the past, so that these things can be done even more in the present and future.
- They can help form the basis for discussions about tricky situations and give the worker confidence to say 'I don't know, what do you

think we should do?' They relieve the worker from needing to know the solution to every problem that comes along and help the worker tap into the ideas and resources of the person who has AS.

References

Ajmal, Y. and Rees, I. (2001) *Solutions in Schools: Creative Applications of Solution Focused Brief Thinking with Young People and Adults.* London: BT Press.

Department of Health (2006) 'Better services for people with an autistic spectrum disorder: A note clarifying current Government policy and describing good practice.' Available at www.dh.gov.uk/Publicationsandstatistics (accessed 6 August 2007).

Edmonds, G. and Worton, D. (2005) *The Asperger Love Guide.* London: Sage Publications/Paul Chapman Publishing.

Edmonds, G. and Worton, D. (2006a) *The Asperger Social Guide.* London: Sage Publications/Paul Chapman Publishing.

Edmonds, G. and Worton, D. (2006b) *The Asperger Personal Guide.* London: Sage Publications/Paul Chapman Publishing.

Hesmondhalgh, M. and Jackson, J. (2006) *Autism, Access and Inclusion on the Front Line: Confessions of an Autism Anorak.* London: Jessica Kingsley Publishers.

Mayer, R.N. (2001) *Asperger Syndrome Employment Workbook.* London: Jessica Kingsley Publishers.

Powell, A. (2002) *Taking Responsibility: Good Practice Guidelines for Services – Adults with Asperger Syndrome.* London: National Autistic Society.

Chapter Six

Seven People and a Social Group

Introduction

What we want to achieve here is the telling of practical stories which illustrate how solution focused approaches can be used with people who have AS. The problem we run into when trying to write this is that we cannot illustrate situations or points any better than by telling what happens in real live clinical sessions, and we can't seem to talk about real live clinical sessions in any great depth without saying things that would identify the person about whom we are talking. Early on we both decided that it would be best to write case stories alongside the people who featured in them. However, this then became a story about them and not necessarily about solution focused brief therapy. So we ended up writing great stories of intrigue, heroism, compromises, mysteries, fires, floods, famine and locusts – but alas, not for this book!

For this section of the book, we have decided that Vicky could write about a few individuals with different needs. In a sense, this then becomes a case study of how Vicky applies solution focused principles to some common and some uncommon situations and we get to talk about more case examples without going into identity-revealing depth on any one person (we hope). Details of the people have been changed, such as gender, age, family composition and so on, while the essence of the clinical issues is kept true to the real situation, in an effort to uphold the integrity of the actual clinical work.

Every problem and every solution comes from Vicky's clinical work. However, things do not always happen as 'cut and dried' as they appear in print. One loses the length of silences, body language, and other aspects of sessional work by writing in this way. Nevertheless, it quickly becomes clear that people with AS are very similar and very different from each other at the same time. We hope that people do not feel exposed by these stories, except of course for Vicky, who is in a position to write about both her external behaviour and her internal states while she is working.

Vicky works with people who do not have AS as well, but we have excluded them from these brief case studies because, well, because this book is about AS.

Sam on probation

Another week begins. After the horses go out, the dog goes in and the cat pleases himself, I am off to see Sam, my first AS person of the week.

Sam was referred to me by his social worker. He has a pretty impressive record as a serial offender with non-violent offences, for which the court also ordered he seek 'counselling'. His probation officer does not know what to do, but the social worker on Sam's support team thought Sam might have AS, so he wonders if I might meet Sam and see whether or not counselling might help. Of course I will, and so this is where I am headed on this wet Monday morning. The rain pelts down even harder when it becomes evident there are no parking places near to the office where I am to meet Sam. Soaked, I drip into reception, where a cheerful woman takes me to the waiting room and introduces me to Sam. She trots up two flights of stairs, Sam makes a rather gallant 'after you' gesture, and I drip, squelch and squeak up after her. As we arrange ourselves in the echoing room, I notice that Sam does not make any eye contact. He sits, somewhat glumly, it appears, with rounded shoulders, hands loosely clasped, and a fixed gaze at the carpet. I bring my chair around and look at him with a dripping smile.

'Not very nice weather this morning. Have you been waiting long for me to arrive?'

'No,' he says, looking at his fingers.

'Well,' I say, 'I guess you know that Richard, your social worker, asked me to see you, but I am a little unclear what it is we ought to talk about. Do you have any ideas?'

Silence.

'Is there anything in particular you hoped we might talk about today?' This is a typical solution focused opening gambit, as I am interested to begin constructing some kind of agenda with Sam for the hour we will spend together. I want to know what will have to happen during our conversation in order for him to feel his time has been well spent.

Silence. (Sam, I think to myself, has not read the solution focused handbook, and does not know the rules!)

I address the uncomfortable and tricky situation of payment, because Sam has to pay for these sessions himself, even though the court has ordered him to get counselling and the social worker has arranged the appointment. He says he is happy to pay me and that he has some money he can use for this purpose. I note that it is unfortunate that the court can require something which is not freely available to him. I think it is tight that the court says he must do this thing, and that he must pay for it, whether or not he finds it useful. He shrugs.

Sam is not particularly forthcoming, but it transpires that he has been arrested for petty theft, flashing, and, oddly, for laughing at the police person when he was questioned about another crime. This last offence was called 'creating public nuisance' or something similar. He has had difficulty with the police on and off since he was sixteen, and he is now almost thirty. At his recent court appearance it was suggested he get yet another psychiatric report to see if he has Asperger Syndrome, which he duly attended. I ask him the outcome of this and he shrugs his shoulders and says 'The man said AS couldn't be diagnosed in adults because they might lie about the symptoms. He says people use AS as a way of avoiding responsibility for their bad behaviour. He says I want to keep re-offending.'

'Ah, yes, well, is he right?'

'Dunno.'

'Well. Me neither.' My head is truly empty on this point as I am waiting for Sam to tell me where our conversation needs to go next. Only Sam doesn't seem to know where it ought to go, so I ask him to tell me a little about himself.

Turns out that Sam was briefly married once but had no children. His wife of 12 months asked him for a divorce about five years ago. Since then he has been living on his own, and some of the problems of offending have come to the fore again. He apparently was a thieving, flashing, public nuisance before he was married, but just a flashing public nuisance after he was married. For the year he was married he did not offend at all. I am interested in this exception to the problem, because whatever was working to keep him out of the criminal justice system then will be worth learning about, but I tuck it away for later discussion so as not to interrupt his story.

Sam says his most recent job was in a supermarket, but he lost this about four years ago in a repeat performance of every other job he has had, and so he is sensibly reluctant to try working again. He tells a familiar tale of employment breakdown because of problems getting along with co-workers. He felt they were making fun of him, and he thought they did not like him very much. Still, even though it was uncomfortable being with his co-workers, he managed to keep going in to work, doing his full shift and not taking any time off sick. I note that this must take extraordinary commitment and strength. He shrugs the observation off so I leave it hanging in the air.

I can see that he is a quiet, gentle man and it seems as though he truly wants to do the right things, but he continues to appear in the wrong places at the wrong time and to make spectacular mistakes reading the social cues of others. He tells of few childhood friends except for one or two boys, one of whom made a career out of stealing and substance abuse. He tells stories about how these boys used to dare him to do things, and says this is how he was first introduced to the criminal justice system. By good fortune he has avoided custodial sentences and he says he knows that if he continues to break the law he may go to jail, and he really doesn't want to do this. He also notes that sometimes it is hard to know exactly when he is and is not breaking the law. He is surprised, as am I, that laughing in the presence of a policeman can get him into such trouble. He says he laughed because he 'was scared s***less and didn't know what to do'. He was surprised to find that he was laughing because he certainly didn't think anything was funny at the time. The police called this a breach of the peace and creating a public nuisance. I am certain there would be a different tale from the policeman involved, because he probably thought Sam was goading him or not taking him seriously by laughing. At this stage, though, I am more interested in the reality that Sam has constructed for himself as opposed to what the policeman might have been thinking.

Sam starts giving me good eye contact about 15 minutes into our session as I ask about how he has coped with this difficult history. He says he visits prostitutes, some of whom take drugs, though he doesn't do this himself. He also used to visit his burglar friend, but this man is now locked up, so he doesn't go and see him. He says he also has 'quirks' that he indulges when he is alone in his home and this offers him some satisfaction and relief.

'How does seeing prostitutes help?' I ask.

'Well, it is nice to have some company,' he says sensibly. 'I like to talk to them, but not all of them want to talk. I can tell when one wants to talk and when one wants to just get it over with.' Because I am listening for strengths and skills, I make a mental note that this is perhaps an indication of empathy or the reading of non-verbal language, which people with AS are not supposed to be able to do.

'I don't suppose many of them find men that actually want to listen to them. You probably come as a surprise in that respect. *Do* you listen to them?' I ask with a little surprise in my voice.

'Oh yes. They are very interesting and there are a few that appreciate the time I take to listen to them. Of course there are others that steal your money too; they tend to talk a little less.' We smile at the understatement.

I ask where he learned to be such a good listener. I am also interested to know how he tells the women who want to talk from the ones who don't, because I note that this will require a little bit of reading signals from them, which people with autism are not supposed to be able to do. He talks much more freely about these things. His eye contact is still unusual in its intensity, in as much as he stares at me, in a spooky kind of way, when talking about something of interest, but he is engaging with me better than he was initially. Also, I notice a smile or two has crept across his face as he talks.

His preferred future is to be 'normal' again. More questioning as to what 'normal' means for him reveals that he wants to have a girlfriend and some other friends with whom he could spend time. He has no friends now, and spends his time either with prostitutes or on his own. He does not see his family any more, though he does remember them on birthdays and at Christmas. Likewise they remember him, but this seems to be the extent of their contact. He says if he had a girlfriend and other friends he would feel he belonged somewhere and he would feel accepted. He also would have someone to help him understand things like getting along with people. He said his wife pretty much took care of social things, and without her he was out of his depth again. He seems surprised that he can still get into as much bother with the police and neighbours now at almost 30 as he used to when he was 16. He says he is worried that he is actually very stupid because of these repeated difficulties, though there are ample signs of intelligence which I am able to notice.

His preferred future also involved getting a job. In answer to my search for details of what worked in his previous employment, he noted that he was actually a good employee in many respects, because he never had time off sick, he was always on time, he worked when he should be working and took breaks when he should be taking breaks. He followed all the rules and learned the job quickly. Things fell apart, he said, when he felt everyone was looking at him and he didn't know what to do. He felt they all knew he was in trouble for flashing or stealing and he became so panicky that he walked out of a few jobs and never came back. His confidence dropped from then onwards, and now he was unable to even go out to a pub for fear of people looking at him, or for fear of naïvely doing something that would attract the attention of the police.

'So,' I summarized, 'your preferred future involves having a partner, having two or three other friends and having a job where you feel happy and secure?'

'Yes. I think that is about it.'

'I guess a good future for you would also mean not having any more involvement with the police?'

'Well, yes…of course.'

'Can you tell me, then, about how the offences have been helpful to you?'

'Er…what?' he asked.

'Well, the stealing only happened a few times between the ages of sixteen and nineteen – is that right?'

'Yeah, that sounds about right.'

'And the public nuisance laughing-at-the-policeman stuff certainly wasn't something you did on purpose?'

'No. No, I still don't understand what went so wrong there.'

'But the flashing has been more long-term than any of those, I notice. I guess my question really is, what do you find helpful about flashing?'

'I never thought about that before.' He takes some time to consider this before he says, 'I think I feel strong and in control when I'm doing it. And I am by myself, so no one is going to confuse me or make fun of me and I am not hurting anyone.'

'OK. So when you flash you feel strong and in control, and confident?'

'Yes, I do. But of course it is wrong to do it and I would rather not do it really, because apparently it does hurt people who see me.'

'Of course, because…because would you say you are pretty much a nice person who would not want to frighten anyone or hurt anyone?'

'Yeah.' Sam looks down at the floor again.

'So a good future would be one in which you would be able to feel strong, in control and confident AND not hurt or frighten anyone at the same time?'

Sam looks up at me with surprise and says simply, 'Yes.'

'Well,' I said, 'that's pretty much my preferred future too. In that respect we are not so different from each other, eh?' We sat in silence for a minute or so because I wanted him to have quiet time to process the idea that he could have strength, control and confidence at the same time as not flashing. I also guessed, but didn't know for sure, that he might appreciate the idea that he and I were more the same than different. Wanting strength, control and confidence is utterly normal and common. The trick is to find these things without hurting or scaring someone else.

I deliberately did not ask Sam questions about frequency or duration of flashing, things that triggered it, and how he reconciled himself to doing something he knew was illegal, and how long he thought he could avoid a custodial sentence if he kept doing this, and so on. I had no interest in establishing a good record of the problems. I had an acute interest in establishing a good record of his successes and strengths along with his hopes for the future.

'Sam,' I asked, 'How on a scale of nought to ten, where zero means that you have absolutely no confidence and ten means you have absolute confidence, how confident are you that you will be able to get this preferred future?'

He thought about this for a long time. Most people do think about this for a long time, as it is an unusual question, really. Finally he said somewhat apologetically, 'About a two, I think.'

'A two?!' I responded. 'Gosh, how come a two and not a one?'

'What?'

'Well, a two suggests that there are a few things you know about that give you a little bit of confidence. I was wondering what those things were?'

'Um. Well, I dunno really,' he said, thinking again. I waited quietly for what seemed a long time. 'Well, I have had a relationship before, and I have had jobs before, so I ought to be able to at least get them again.'

'Yes,' I said. 'I think you probably can do that again. What else gives you confidence?'

'Um.' The clock ticked darkly while he was thinking in silence. 'Well, I really do want to leave all this police business behind. I really do want to feel normal again.'

'Ah, excellent. So you feel you are really motivated to do something different – that is, something out of your present routine – in order to get the future you want?'

'Yes. Yes, I think so,' Sam said with a little smile.

As we progressed through towards the end of the session, I said to Sam that I knew he felt people didn't like him, but I simply could not understand why this would be so. I noticed that he took care about how he looked, that he listened when I talked, that he seemed genuine in what he said, and other positive aspects of his character. Sam was silent for a long time and I saw that he had tears in his eyes. He said he didn't know anyone could tell those things about him, and if they were true, why was he in such a mess?

'I don't know,' I said. 'I was wondering the same thing myself.' I wanted to reinforce here that we were working together to understand the situation and that I had no expert answers to give him. I think in my previous problem focused life as a behaviour therapist I probably would have pointed out that he was in such a mess because he insisted on doing a hurtful and illegal behaviour. With my experience working in a solution focused way I know that nothing is quite this simplistic, and I know that Sam and I together will arrive at a satisfactory way forward, even if we never understand exactly why he keeps offending.

He said he wanted to make another appointment, and I suggested that, as he had said reading the intentions of others was anxiety-provoking for him, we meet in a public place such as a pub that was open in the afternoon. That way we could practise noticing if other people were looking at him, and we could keep a check on his anxiety about being in a public place. He hesitated in agreeing to this, but brightened when he thought of a pub in which he felt comfortable, and agreed. We made an appointment to do this, and we both went out into the rain.

Despite getting wet again on the way to my car, my heart smiled a bit about this lovely man and his genuine confusion about how he ended up in 'such a mess'. This confusion is understandable, given the way his mind processes information in a linear, factual way. He seemed to be making large decisions on the basis of tiny details, such as 'when people look at me, they do not like me' and then spending his life living by this huge decision. He seemed surprised that we did not talk about offences, and he was mildly uncomfortable with the positive aspects of his character that I noticed. Still, there was, I felt, huge capacity for changing his fixed beliefs and a real possibility of him attaining his preferred future.

Phil: the quiet man

Next, a long wet drive to another town to see a nineteen-year-old boy who was just recovering from a car accident. He had broken his leg and his wrist. His family were worried that he wrecked the car on purpose because he no longer wanted to live. This is what he told the psychiatrist when he moved from the acute medical ward to the psychiatric rehabilitation unit. His parents were told by professionals that Phil could not express his emotion well enough to benefit from counselling, so, apart from medication, there was little they could do for him. He was ill enough to qualify for supported living, however, so he moved into a flat with a staff team to help him. He shared the staff with eight other residents of the apartment complex. His parents suspected that he had AS, but did not know whether a diagnosis would help or hinder him. Their preferred future for my work with him was simply to 'talk to him and form an opinion about his mental health and the risk of him trying to kill himself'.

The first time I saw Phil was four weeks previously, and so this was my second visit with him. He did not want to see me any more frequently than once a month, because of the expense. (His parents were paying and he was worried about them being able to afford this, though they said I ought not to worry about it.) He also wanted to leave a little time between visits because he might not have anything to talk to me about if he saw me more frequently. During my first visit I firmly believed he was taking too much medication because he seemed to have great difficulty concentrating, difficulty forming words, difficulty thinking what it was he wanted to say, and he looked impossibly sleepy. To my surprise, when I checked with the staff after my first conversation with him, he was taking *no* medication at all! The first visit was quite hard work and I was not particularly looking forward to this second visit, as I was unsure how to go about helping Phil to connect with me. We had agreed at the end of the first session that it would be easier to *do* something when I next came, rather than just talk. I said I would bring some things we could do, and so I brought my box of tricks (mostly art materials) up to his flat on this rainy Monday. I was pinning my hopes on these arty-crafty materials because I didn't know what else I might do to stimulate some conversation with him. I don't mind this level of 'empty-headedness', however, because if I listen well enough the client will come up with ways for us to engage with each other.

I was simply amazed when I entered his flat on my second visit. He had not only remembered our arrangement to do something, he had, with staff help, organized a jigsaw puzzle on the table ready for my arrival. He smiled upon greeting me, remembered my name and asked me if I wanted to make myself a drink. (He was still mostly immobile from his various fractures.) I asked him questions about his choice of puzzle – wildlife – discussed his experiences with animals and talked about things he liked to do. He still struggled to put full sentences together, but his eye contact and attention were magnificent in comparison to our first meeting. I commented on this and ask what differences he had noticed in himself between my first visit and this one. This is a common solution focused question, asking for between-session changes. He couldn't really think of any, so I said last time I was worried because his thoughts seemed so 'disjointed' and he looked so sleepy. He smiled and said sometimes he was like that when he did not know which way a conversation was going to go. He said he only saw me that first time because his family insisted, not because he wanted to. He said he had never got along with other psychologists and he didn't really think I could help him. He said he had decided now that I was OK and not really like a normal psychologist, so I could come back again. (I knew my abnormality would come in handy one day!)

Well, it was my turn to be speechless because I didn't know any of that, and I told him so. We spent the hour chatting and puzzle working, and at the end he said that was one of the best sessions he had ever had. I honestly had no idea what happened in the session that made him call it 'the best', because mainly he talked, while I listened and commented on what I thought I heard him say. He clarified what I heard, I summarized, and then we went on to talk about something else. When I asked what difference he thought our good session would make to him or others, he said his mum would notice him being more talkative and the staff would notice he was hungry for his lunch, which he usually isn't. Gosh…I love this guy! I will have some more clients like this please!

As I was packing the car, ready to move on, I reflected that during this second session Phil and I had not attempted to talk about emotions, or to use feeling words, because these in the first session had seemed to be foreign to him. My observations to him were based on what I saw him doing right at the moment, which was something he seemed able to grasp. For example, I asked how he could so quickly find the right piece of the puzzle. Was it by colour? Size? Shape? These were questions he could work with, and to my great relief he made the effort to converse quite successfully this time. If I had not asked, I would never have known the complex thinking that was behind his behaviour, though I could easily have found a chapter in a textbook to give me a theory about why people would not engage with a therapist. At least by listening to his view I was working with the facts as he saw them, rather than a theory that some very smart person writing a book guessed about.

I wondered whether or not focusing on things he liked, giving him plenty of choice about when to see me and what we ought to do, and not directing the conversation onto whether or not he was depressed enough to kill himself might have helped him to become so comfortable with me so quickly. One of the advantages of any kind of brief therapy is that working relationships are established quickly, and I feel that solution focused work gives me a great structure for doing this. I was able to come to the second session with no 'shoulds', 'oughts' or 'musts' about what *he* had to do, though I did have some absolutes about what *I* needed to do: 'I should listen as hard as I can', 'I ought to find out what he wants from our work together', and 'I must converse with him on an equal footing'. I had no expectations about what *he* needed to talk about or accomplish at this second session. Given my experience of the first session, I would have been pleased if he had only managed to stay awake and maintain attention during my second session! To actually have a two-way conversation with him was an unexpected bonus.

Prior to my using solution focused work, I would have tried to tie his behaviour in the last session to words like 'resistance', 'fear', or some other emotion word. I probably would have insisted we talk, rather than agreeing to do an activity, even though just doing an activity would give me lots of time to notice strengths, attention span, likes, dislikes, abilities, motor coordination, ways of dealing with frustration, asking for help or advice, and countless other useful strengths and skills. I doubtless would have imposed my theory about how thoughts, feelings and behaviours are connected, and how we need to know how each is influencing the other in order to 'be happy' again. I do not think this would have worked with Phil.

Fergus-of-the-fixed-views

Next on the list was Fergus-of-the-fixed-views, whose claim to fame was having more diagnoses than hot dinners; some professionally given and some self-conferred. I had been seeing Fergus for about six sessions and was exhausted after each of them. Fergus lived alone in a family-owned bungalow with no staff or family support. According to his various conditions, he qualified for support from every conceivable team in both the NHS and Social Services, yet at the time I met him he had no one helping him on any kind of routine basis. I was being funded by a local primary care trust as part of interim work I was doing to cover for another psychologist's maternity leave. Fergus had one friend who lived 70 miles away, and problems enough to fox all the King's horses and all the King's men. It was hard for me to know where to start each session, but Fergus always knew where to begin and end each session, such that the sixth session was very much like the first session, with an increasing sense from me that we were not actually making any progress. Yet Fergus kept agreeing to see me, so I guessed that something must be useful about my visits.

Fergus, living alone as he did, had developed unchallenged theories about everything. He knew why people didn't like him, he knew why services wouldn't provide him with support, he knew why credit companies hassled him, he knew why he didn't have a job, and he knew why he was so socially isolated. The reason for all these things was that no one wanted to give him exactly what he asked for, and I mean *exactly* what he asked for. Themes that emerged from our discussions were similar to 'If X [insert any team or individual name] is going to provide me with a service, then they will have to change their ideas and give me some respect.' Only the thing is, X actually doesn't *have* to change anything if X doesn't want to, but Fergus simply did not accept this point of view. Other people *must* change and then I will be 'OK'. He tried to change a few things about me too, such as stopping me from clicking my pen, though he didn't insist I do everything his way, or make any unreasonable requests of me at all. He did seem to treat me a little differently than he did most other professionals.

So a predominant thing I noticed about Fergus was that his preferred future involved staying exactly how he was, while everyone else around him changed their ways. Our conversations were heavy with 'stuckness' because he refused to bend in his opinions and views of 'The Way Things Had to Be'. Fergus said he had a Personality Disorder. He also had Attention Deficit Disorder. He had Myasthenia Gravis. He had Bi-polar Depression. He had Chronic Fatigue Syndrome, because he'd seen a TV programme about it and recognized the symptoms in himself. He doubted that he had AS though, and if he did, he said, it did not affect him as much as the other things he had, so he wanted services to ignore the AS and just give him something for the stress, depression and physical ailments. He required a walking stick, special creams and ointments, a perching stool, and lots of medical/psychological assessments. He was allergic to lots of fabric and sunshine. He couldn't sleep. He sacked the physiotherapist because they would not offer five minutes of pain-relieving zaps from a machine when he asked them. They said they could only give him three minutes of zaps so they parted company. He was socially isolated, and felt he could be dead in his flat and no one would know for days. He demanded an emergency cord be installed in his home. He had a flair-up of his chronic fatigue out of office hours and made a complaint because NHS Direct would not send a physician to his bedside immediately. Because credit card companies and banks helpfully provided him with lots of credit, he was tens of thousands of pounds in debt, yet felt he required a new computer system. He wanted me to initiate the complaints procedure against a well-known shop because they refused him credit when they checked his credit reference and found it unsatisfactory. Dearie me, our sessions were fast-paced and furious.

My game plan had been to hold grimly onto solution focused principles even though I was mentally buffeted and battered at each session. There was a strong feeling of having to do fancy footwork, dodge, thrust and parry, keeping alert every second of every minute of every long hour I spent with him. Fergus wanted things to be different and by golly, he was prepared to fight everyone he met to ensure people knew what he wanted. And he was no wimp, as I quickly discovered. He could out-manoeuvre, out-think and out-distance me without so much as breaking a sweat. Still we persisted together.

Local services had actually tried to respond several times, but it seems they found it impossible to work within Fergus-of-the-fixed-views' framework. I think it was the solution focused principles of using the client's own language, steadfastly believing that the client is cooperating the best they can at any given moment, and believing absolutely (with the faith of a child?) that people know what will and will not work for them. These were the main safety belts with which I secured myself when I sat on the settee to begin our discussions. The safety belts didn't stop me rocking with anxiety, which I renamed 'deep concentration' when Fergus asked me in a demandingly loud voice why I was rocking.

So, here I was for the seventh time, walking up the drive to his bungalow. 'Do you have any good news for me?' he asked before I had finished closing the door behind me.

I never quite knew what answer he wanted when he asked this. Sometimes I just said 'no', sometimes I said 'News? What about?' and sometimes I said 'Yes. I didn't get run over today.' His response was the same each time. Hands on hips, he rolled his eyes heavenward and said 'You know what I mean' (I didn't, honestly), 'have you heard anything from the bank/ doctor/psychiatrist/neurologist/ear, nose and throat man/social worker/mechanic/plumber, etc.' Never was I able to answer this affirmatively. Once I tried to answer this question before he asked it, just to see what would happen, but he carried on as if I hadn't said anything and asked the question anyway. This made me wonder if, somehow, the purpose of the question wasn't to ask a question at all. The purpose of the question might be something like signalling the start of the session, or helping him to organize his thoughts, or something else useful for him. I did ask him once why he always asked me that question first and he stopped stock-still (he always paced while he talked) and said, 'You know why I ask that,' and before I could follow this up I fell down another hole with him and got involved in the familiar scenario where yet another unsuspecting person had done him wrong.

'Have you got any good news for me?' I countered on this seventh visit. 'Tell me what's been better since my last visit.' (Please, oh please, I added in my mind, please tell me something has got better...)

Alas, no, there was no improvement in society's behaviour in which we could jointly rejoice, and certainly there was no change in his own behaviour, but that wasn't under discussion anyway, was it? Our seventh exchange went much like our first exchange.

'Gosh, Fergus. How do you manage to cope with all these things going wrong?' It is a genuine question on my part because I would have been crushed long ago living with his interpretation of life.

'You know how I cope!' He always credited me with knowing the most amazing things, which I swear I did not know. Perhaps I ought to have felt flattered by that instead of mildly confused.

'Remind me.'

'I get very depressed, I don't sleep, I cry every night, I want to kill myself, I become ill! Wouldn't you?'

'Aye, Fergus. I probably would at that. Tell me then, if you and I together could do just the right things and fix even one of these situations, what would be better for you?'

'I wouldn't be socially isolated for one thing. I would have people coming in to support me. People that listened to me and did what I wanted.'

'So if we found the right people who could listen to you and do what you wanted, what would be different about you?'

'Let's put it this way, Vicky,' he said as if talking to a child, 'I would be happy.' Then he masterfully swept me off to discuss the wrongdoings of someone else. I tried very hard to keep a focus on the detail of what would be better if we did the right things, but he was stronger in personality and fleeter of thought than me, and my brain ended up (again) in a sweaty heap gasping for air. I was grateful during these times for his continuing monologue because I could do a mental Formula One pit stop, change the wheels and grease up the gasping brain ready to try something different in the next part of the session.

'What is it about you, Fergus, that allows you to cope with all this isolation?' I asked. Again, as with all solution focused questions, this one was born out of genuine interest, because this man somehow had built up the strength of an army.

'I cope because I have to because no one will help me...'

I jump in quick here because I feel him dragging me into another dark hole of who is not doing what he wants them to do. A bit recklessly, perhaps, I ask 'Why? Why do you have to cope? Why not stop coping?'

Again he rolls his eyes up to the gods and says 'Let's put it this way, if I didn't cope every day I would be dead by now. I would be dead if I didn't have some hope that we would get this sorted some day.'

'You have hope?!' I say with too much astonishment in my voice. 'Tell me [please], what gives you hope that we can sort this out?'

'I have to have hope! That's all I got left!'

'Yes. I can see that. And I am glad you have hope. I was just wondering if you could point to anything that gives you that hope? Do you think, for example, that services actually want to help you out? Do you think that they would help if they knew what to do? Maybe?'

'I think they would help if I just accepted whatever they did. That's what I think. I don't think people like it when I tell them what I want them to do. I think I am just supposed to take whatever they give and like it.'

Ah. Yes. 'Actually Fergus, I think you are right there. I think people are used to providing support in a certain way, using certain rules, and that they may be surprised when you ask for something different. Which is better, do you think: a) to accept any kind of help so that you are not socially isolated or b) to refuse any help because it is not exactly how you want it?'

'It is better to refuse help that I don't want. How can people expect me to use help if I don't understand why it's being done, how long it is going to be given or who is going to be giving it? Yet no one can ever give me answers to these questions. People think I can do lots more things than I can actually do, you know. People do not believe I need help to get my groceries in, even though I tell them that I need help. People don't believe I need help to clean or organize my flat, or that I need help changing light bulbs, or doing the simplest of things. I am caught between appearing competent, so that I constantly have to prove how incompetent I am, but I can't prove it to the satisfaction of services. And that doesn't feel good!'

'Well. You are, it seems to me, in a pretty crap situation really.' What Fergus says makes sense, yet it doesn't work to get him the future that he wants. He is in a common trap between services that is all too familiar to people with autism.

He laughs. 'I like that you are so straight-talking. Other people try to convince me that services do listen and do provide what I want and are...what's the word...person centred. But they are not. At least not where I am concerned. I have to fight all the time, and I don't want to fight all the time, but I don't want to give up and just accept less than what I deserve either.'

'Hell. It must be hell, eh?'

'Yes. It is actually.'

'So then. I don't know what to do to get you the services that you want. And so far you're saying that what you've been trying to do, which is in essence to force people to give you want you want, you're saying that that isn't working, so we need to do something different, only we don't know exactly what to do. Would you say that's right?'

Laughing again: 'I would say that's a pretty honest summary, yes.'

'Well, never mind for the moment what it is that we do, let's pretend that we accidentally do absolutely the right thing during the next week. What will be the first thing you notice that tells you things are improving?' This is a version of a simple preferred future question that is kind of related to the Miracle Question. These types of questions have not been successful in generating detail of what Fergus wants to be different in his life, so if this simplified general question achieves results, I might then decide to go for more detail.

'Let's put it this way, I wouldn't be so sick all the time.'

What?! Do my ears deceive me or has Fergus just given me a big clue as to how to reverse the growing list of complaints and ailments? 'You mean if we were to do just the right thing, you would start to feel physically better and perhaps not need to see your GP so much?'

'Possibly, but that is too much to hope for just now.'

Again Fergus has given me an idea here about how these frequent detours down the black hole of complaints about other people are his best way of cooperating with me. I can now check out with him whether or not he redirects the conversation back to these complaints because imagining a future without all these complaints is too scary or 'too much to hope for just now'. If this is the case, I can be a little easier about these diversions because they represent no more than a bit of breathing space which Fergus is giving himself. I would check out with him whether or not the time we spend identifying exactly what would be different in his new life without the problems will increase as he gains more confidence that he can actually achieve this new life. From experience I have learned that it is a far more pleasant and productive conversation to talk about increasing something positive, like confidence, than it is to keep harping on decreasing something negative, like complaints about various and sundry people.

And you know, for all that he exercises my mental capacity, and for all his bluster and 'let's put it this way', I actually like the man. I feel very inadequate when I am with him, and I can see that he is a strong, worthwhile character who has, in the main, treated me with respect. That said, I am still relieved when our time is over (he prefers two-hour sessions rather than the more typical one-hour sessions, naturally) and I can slope back to the quiet of my car. I say quiet, but I actually can hear bits of my brain sloshing about.

I start my drive home and wonder if there are any signs of small successes with dear Fergus. I ask the dozing therapist in my mind what she will notice when Fergus is one little step better. The mental therapist wakes and says, 'When he lets you finish a sentence without interrupting; when he has a conversation in quieter tones rather than cross-examining everything you say; when he starts a session saying he's had a good week…' *Stop*! I tell her, I only wanted one… Still I note that I did get to finish a few sentences today and I did learn that the many and varied diversions may be fulfilling an important need to keep the pace of change slow. And, I note with both humour and despair, seven sessions is more than any other therapist has ever lasted with him. I have to trust him if I am to stay solution focused.

I finish my day at home, answering emails and phone calls, and getting some much needed 'fur' therapy from my animals. They never once say 'Let me put it this way…', which I very much appreciate.

Seth's team meeting

I was invited to attend a planning meeting where I was to summarize my handful of sessions with a man, Seth, who had been flummoxing local services. Meetings are not my strong point, really, because I fiddle and wiggle a lot and can be quietly disruptive if the meeting lasts more than 20 minutes, which all meetings do as a matter of universal law. Typically of a person with AS, I find the things I have to contribute to the meeting vitally interesting, but I occasionally struggle to maintain concentration when other people are talking. The phrase that has been applied to me, aptly I think, is 'eccentric but useful'.

So off I go to the meeting. Prepared, I am pleased to say, with a written report of our work, plus some recommendations for further work which Seth and I had discussed at our last meeting. I am looking forward to seeing Seth and meeting his family.

A police officer, social worker, psychologist, and community mental health nurse come for the meeting, along with Seth, his mother, his father and his brother. The turnout is good, I think, which I hope conveys to Seth that there are quite a few people interested in getting support right for him. Even though I am not the official host of the meeting, I offer to get brews for everyone while the social worker does some last-minute photocopying. I like being helpful in practical ways like this.

Once settled, everyone is silent while they read the report that Seth and I have written – except for me, of course; because I wrote the thing, I don't need to read it now, so I gently and quietly bebop around in my twirly chair and rhyme words in my head. I am then asked to summarize the report, which I do by talking mainly to Seth, just to double-check that what I have written and summarized is indeed representative of the work we have done. Seth contributes too, and I am reminded again of what a charming, kind and generous character he is. I start by turning to his family and saying something like, 'You must be very proud of Seth because despite some differences in how he processes information, he has held down a job, and managed many difficult situations with grace and dignity. Clearly you as his family have done many things right and your support of him shows in his character.' What's that then? Does Dad have allergies or is that a tear in his eye? I make a mental note of it but don't comment.

What happens then is that Seth and his family and I have a conversation about what ought to happen next to support Seth. The others there do contribute, and it is clear they have known Seth much longer than I have. I did not realize there was this lengthy history between them all, but then there was no particular reason why I ought to know either. I had been told by some of the professionals present that Seth's family seemed odd and 'difficult', and I remembered this as I talked with them, because I found them reasonable people who wanted the best for their son/brother.

I especially liked the brother because he clearly knew Seth well and he seemed very good at reading Seth's body language throughout the meeting. We did, as well-meaning people tend to do, leap straight for solutions like 'How about attending this group?' or 'What about a job doing this thing or that thing?' whereas his brother brought us back to the details of Seth's life that also needed attention. He felt that something like ten of hours of support per week from a relaxed support worker would be helpful in just helping Seth establish some daily routine in his life. He talked about the importance of eating well, of enjoying a trip to the shop to get groceries, about the importance of someone cueing Seth to talk to people in the shop and to 'come out of himself' a bit more. I thought he sounded very sensible and on track.

I also liked how Seth's family seemed naturally talented at seeing the glass as half full instead of half empty. That is, they saw Seth's considerable strengths rather than the list of things he couldn't do, and they wanted to know how we could help him build on these strengths rather than focus too much on the problems. In short, I enjoyed my conversation with Seth and his family and learned from the contributions of others present as well. In the main, the whole meeting had a positive feel to me.

Father made a point to thank me after the meeting because he appreciated my positive focus, he said. It was genuinely my pleasure, no thanks was necessary, but it felt nice just the same. I thought the meeting went well, and I was in a whistling good mood really.

Seth and his family left the meeting room, and I must say I was completely stunned by what happened next. The professionals in the room began to talk about how difficult the meeting was. They felt we had gone 'completely off at a tangent' and that we did not have a real grasp of how serious Seth's behaviour was. People who admittedly had much more experience with the family felt that the family were out of touch with the reality of Seth's behaviour problems. They also had pointed remarks to make about my summary of our work together, saying that some of the things written in it, which had been remarks of Seth's, were simply not true. Gosh. I felt as though I had attended a different meeting than they had.

This group were insisting that Seth presented a serious risk to himself and, I guess, to other people, though the nature of these risks was not exactly clear to me. They worried about his family being involved in his care plan, because he was an adult and as such the family didn't need to know about his care plans and assessment summaries. As I say, I was stunned at the apparent differences in our interpretations of what happened during the meeting. I asked for specifics because I was worried I had missed something important.

'What?!' I asked. 'What did we talk about that was off on a tangent?'

'Well, that bit about having a daily routine and shopping and everything. What Seth needs is a job, and to have a little pressure applied so that he stays out of trouble and does something worthwhile with his life.'

'Oh. Now you see,' I said trying to explain myself, 'I thought those ideas were actually good ones, because getting a routine established for Seth would probably be really helpful, and people with AS may need cueing to have a regular conversation with a shop assistant.'

Well, they would have none of it. They recited all the services that had already been tried with Seth. He has had job coaches. He has had CBT several times and made no improvement. The social worker highlighted the number of arguments he had had with Seth about how wrong his behaviour was, and he was worried that Seth wasn't really interested in changing his behaviour. In fact, his lack of motivation to change his behaviour was the problem, they reckoned.

Odd, that, I thought. Our interventions don't work and somehow Seth is blamed for that. I said in what I hoped was a helpful tone, 'All that means is that we haven't got the support right yet. You have done a good job trying things, and we know a little bit about what doesn't work now, which is helpful. I guess I would be inclined to listen to Seth and to his family about what things will work. They have, after all survived this long so they will know a thing or two about what does and doesn't work.' This is almost straight from the solution focused book. I was working from the philosophy that people know best what does and does not make sense to them. Also, just by surviving difficulties, people have developed skills and strengths that we need to notice and name, then bring to bear on solving current problems. If we don't acknowledge these skills, they will be overlooked and we will be missing out on valuable resources. I was also thinking that if our professional 'programmes' for people don't work, maybe the programmes weren't right and it isn't actually the client's fault. This isn't a hanging offence for a professional, so long as they learn from it what does and doesn't work. It is simply silly to insist that, maybe because we are professionals, what we suggest will work if only the client tries hard enough, or is good enough, or whatever. I am sure though, that that is not what these professionals were thinking because, held up to the light of day, that thinking is kind of crazy.

I left that meeting genuinely wondering what had just happened and where it all went wrong. I felt heartened that while the family and Seth were there, a positive note was struck, and at the same time I remained doubtful that relaxed, positive support would be purchased and put in to help Seth. Sadly, I was now out of the picture, so the family and the lovely Seth would sink or swim without me. I did slip them my card along with the new Department of Health document 'Better services for people with autistic spectrum disorder' (Department of Health 2006), so they went away with some information in case it came in handy.

Paddy the policeman

My next appointment of the day was with a constable, who had self-diagnosed AS, and his partner. They had referred themselves to me both for a formal confirmation of the diagnosis and for some ideas as to how to maintain their relationship, which was plagued by a one-sided lack of emotion, poor communication and an over-zealous mother (mother-in-law for the partner). They were charming company and showed evidence of well-established senses of humour. A formal diagnosis appointment usually takes a minimum of two hours, and their preferred outcome for their expenditure of time and money included this formal diagnosis plus some ideas about how to repair their relationship. I suggested we set our limit at two hours and I would juggle both aims as best I could. We would assess how the content of the meeting was going about halfway through. As it transpired, many of the diagnostic questions could not be answered because they required information from someone who had known the good policeman when he was very young, and some of the questions did not require a great deal of explanation or discussion because this couple had done their homework and understood the nature of the information needed. I was able to confirm the diagnosis, with the caveat that I did not have any corroborating evidence that the social and imaginative differences had been present since early childhood, but that on balance it seemed that AS would be an appropriate diagnosis.

Issues of how to repair, then maintain, a good relationship, however, were much trickier. Paddy the policeman was prone to flat, factual and simplified statements such as 'I don't love my mother', which he had boldly told his mother a few weeks back. He did not want her to visit him, and he wasn't going to visit her, and he very much wanted her out of his life. As I understood the situation, Mum could not reconcile how her son could say that, so she reasoned that her son's wife, Cruella (not her real name), was behind her banishment from the family. The resulting emails, texts, phone calls and letters had led Paddy to experience extreme stress and had actually made him wonder whether or not he loved his wife now. He said he was confused by things his wife said about his mother and vice versa, and he didn't know how to make the arguments stop. He did not want to discuss the situation any more at all, but Cruella was so distressed by his mother that she wanted some obvious support from her husband. Paddy didn't know what it was she wanted him to do, and was noticing some disturbing similarities between his mother and his wife just at the moment.

Policeman Paddy had some strong opinions about how people ought to cope with anxiety. He felt that they needed to 'get to the root' of the problems, eliminate the root and then get on with things. He did not agree with the taking of anti-depressant medication, which often seems to help people with AS, because he felt that was not excising the root of the problem at all. Both his mother and his wife were taking them, and he felt that this was making the situation worse instead of better.

'So you would like to get at the "root" of what is wrong?' I asked.

'Well, yes,' Paddy said, 'because only then can you proceed to do the right thing. I don't want to be going on like this for months, I want the situation resolved.'

'Ah,' I said, 'if the situation were solved, what would be different for you?'

Paddy looked at me as though I had just spoken ancient words of witchcraft. 'What do you mean, what would be better? Clearly I would not be feeling like this. Clearly I would not need to come to you. Life would be quieter.'

'And for you?' I asked the suffering Cruella. 'What would you notice about Paddy if the situation was resolved?'

She smiled and said, 'Paddy would not go straight to the garage (where he's fixing an old car) when he gets home from work.'

I was noticing that these two, in common with lots of other people I see, were describing their preferred future in terms of what would *not* be happening instead of what *would* be happening. The absence of a problem is not necessarily a solution, however. Paddy not going directly to his garage does not necessarily mean that he would automatically be doing something better. Not 'feeling like this', as the policeman said, does not necessarily mean feeling better. I was keen to try and understand what they thought would be happening, rather than what would not. Paddy had already given me one clue as he said, 'Life would be quieter.'

'Paddy, if life were quieter, do you think you would do something different, rather than going to work on your car, when you get home from work?' I asked.

'Possibly,' he said. 'If I knew that Cruella wasn't going to ask me questions and...need me so much, it would be easier to be around her.'

'Cruella, would that be a sign that things are getting better, if Paddy spent more time with you when he got home?' This was what she implied earlier, but she didn't actually say that this was what she wanted.

'Yes,' she said. 'If we had a meal together in the evening, that would be better.'

'What time?'

'What?'

'What time of day would you have your evening meal?' They had to discuss this briefly between themselves and it transpired that he was most often home by about 7:30.

'And, in order for you to think things are getting a little better, would you have to have dinner together every night of the week?' Again, they had a short discussion about this and went through the other commitments they had during the week. They settled on one night for now, a Tuesday night.

'And we know, I guess, that in order to do this as well as possible, Paddy needs to know that you won't be asking him questions or "needing" him so much, Cruella. Paddy, how will you know if Cruella is needing you the right amount?'

'I don't know,' Paddy said as he shifted in his chair. I noted that Paddy appeared unable to even think about things that did not have a right and wrong answer, and decided not to pursue this at this moment, in order to finish identifying the detail of what was required for them to notice a small measure of success.

'Cruella, do you have any ideas as to what you and Paddy might talk about, that you think might make him less anxious or worried about you needing him?'

'Well, that's a funny thing for you to say, Paddy,' Cruella said. 'I am not sure what you think I need you so much for...'

'I think that because you keep asking me what I am going to do about my mother's phone calls. You keep asking me if I think she really doesn't like you. You keep asking me what you should do about this or that or the other thing and I don't know!' Paddy interrupted with emotion. 'You ask and ask and ask until I have to get away.'

'So,' I said, 'what would either of you rather talk about?' The room was silent save for the ticking clock and the tapping of Cruella's fingernails.

'The weather?' I offered hopefully. 'News of the day? Sport? The number of speeding tickets given out in a typical week? Sex? Drugs? Rock'n'roll?...'

They both smiled. We proceeded to talk about what things interested both of them, and it transpired that they both quite liked to read popular science magazines that could be bought at the local supermarket. These magazines contained short articles about new developments in healthcare, physics, astronomy, and various topics. We eventually agreed that Cruella would buy the new issues of one of the magazines every other week, and she would highlight two articles that they could discuss over dinner on Tuesday evening. When they looked sceptical at this idea, I further suggested she start the conversation by saying 'It says here...', and then proceed to discuss the article. The final caveat I gave was that articles about killing mothers-in-law, disposal of the elderly, voodoo for relatives and adverts for nursing home care were forbidden topics of dinner discussion. We agreed that after dinner, Paddy could retreat to the garage if he wanted to. The rest of the week they could carry on as they wished, and it was thus that they went on their way.

What started out as 'I wish she would shut up' and 'I wish he would listen' turned into one dinner a week with a pre-set topic of conversation. This solution came from their very own lips, as I would never have come up with this as a 'treatment' based on psychological theory. I was very optimistic that one night would turn into two nights and that they would then live more or less happily every after. They made no return visit so I felt I gave them the very best I could for a one-shot deal. Though I would very much like to know how they are now, sometimes one shot is all you get.

Marge in Management

Next visit just around the corner was another team meeting, this time with the manager of a domiciliary care service, the team leader of a house for two men with autism, and the social worker for the men. One of the men had been referred to me by the manager a few days previously because his behaviour was getting out of control and she didn't know what to do. I recall a little despondent feeling when the referral was made, because this particular manager had historically made many referrals for all the people who lived within her catchment area. I had not heard from her in quite a while, though the old tickle in my tummy returned as soon as I heard her voice. She asked that I meet with her and a few others before I made an appointment to see the man at his home.

I arrived and was duly given refreshments and a seat before the familiar litany began. She listed what sounded like every difficult behaviour that one man could do. I mainly drank my cup of tea, nodded, and made little noises to indicate my sympathy with her situation. I used the standard questions of 'What would be different if I did the right thing?' and 'What gives you confidence that anything I do will make any difference?' and a few other things. I guess about an hour went by and I still did not have a clear, detailed idea of what it was she wanted me to do, nor what she would notice, assuming I could actually do what she wanted. She mentioned vague things – that the main problem was that the direct care staff were not working consistently, were not following her advice, and were not keeping good records. I felt a bit stuck, so I did what I always do when I feel stuck and I asked a scaling question. 'Marge (for that was the manager's name), on a scale of nought to ten where zero is absolutely no confidence at all and ten is absolute confidence, how confident are you that this situation will improve?'

To my utter astonishment she announced loudly, 'Five'.

'A five?! Gosh! You are halfway there! What gives you such a high level of confidence?'

She smiled and said, 'I didn't think a five was very high.'

'Nevertheless, something is giving you quite a lot of confidence that the staff will respond in the right way for this gentleman. What gives you such confidence?'

'Well,' she said, 'the staff truly have Stephen's best interests at heart, and they are actually a very experienced staff group. They do want things to be better for him.'

'That's excellent!' I said. I asked the team leader her opinion, because she worked with the staff in the home. She agreed with Marge's assessment and said that the staff actually knew what to do in order to prevent Stephen's challenging behaviour, and that most of the time he didn't challenge them at all. Marge was surprised at this because the records do not reflect this. She was only getting incident reports, so she was only collecting information on the things that were not working very well. The social worker also received these reports, and together they decided that the staff team needed to do something different. That is why they called me.

'So Marge, I am impressed with your observation, that everyone agrees is accurate, that the staff group have Stephen's best interests at heart. How did you know that?'

Marge proceeded to tell me several stories of things she had heard or witnessed that had gone well in the house for Stephen. He had been able to go on a long weekend trip for the first time, he had re-established contact with his mum, he had started going to a social group and he was looking at college courses for next term. The team leader added detail to Marge's statements and the second half of the two-hour meeting had an entirely different feel to it. It transpired that what the manager needed was for the staff team to write down the care plan in enough detail so that she and everyone else knew exactly how to respond if they were with Stephen. She accepted that most of the staff knew how to interact with him, but she needed all the staff to know, and she needed it written down. The team leader said she knew the staff could do this, and she said she would have a team meeting, plus meet with Stephen and his key worker and get a detailed care plan written up. I asked when she thought I ought to go to the house and, again to my astonishment, she suggested that might not be needed, so she would ring me in a month's time to let me know what had happened. Unexpectedly, this turned into a one-off meeting with a very pleasant outcome. This was a first for Marge and for me.

Ginger

Ginger is a 35-year-old woman living with her parents who are, in my estimation, more active and fit than retired people have a right to be. They seem to be involved in looking after the neighbourhood, grandchildren and people at church, as well as their own four children. I was asked to see Ginger because after a childhood, adolescence and early adult life as a compliant, quiet, accommodating person, she was becoming aggressive towards her family. People were being hit and things were being broken. The local NHS service did not feel she could be supported from the learning disability service because she was not 'learning disabled enough' and the mental health services did not feel they could offer her support because she was 'not mentally ill enough'. Honestly, if only Ginger could abide by the service rules, eh? In any case, she was being seen by a psychiatrist who had no experience in autism, or learning disabilities. Apart from his medical input, she was not receiving any support from local services when I first met her. At the time of my visit today, however, she had been introduced to a support worker from the Adult Social Services Team on a few occasions.

Ginger had been taking a medication for a number of years that had eventually damaged her liver. This medication seemed to help her think more clearly and to move on from mental obsessions so as to be able to interact fairly well with other people. The medication had to be stopped and a string of other medications were tried, but Ginger felt ill on all of them, so the psychiatrist was left perplexed as to what to try next. Selective serotonin reuptake inhibitors (SSRIs) have been shown to help some people with AS who have obsessions or are highly anxious, but these medications do take a little time to be fully effective. Often when first taking them, a person feels unwell for a week or so. For people who have a poor concept of time, or difficulty in communication, it is difficult to understand that this is temporary, but it is worth persevering for this short period to see if the medication does indeed help them in the long run.

As medications were tried, we were not sure if Ginger was experiencing common side effects or if she was really too ill to take the medication. Over the course of trying one medication, she woke her parents in the middle of the night, saying she thought she had Down's Syndrome and that she wasn't really their daughter. She was always very tearful and her stomach was always upset. She stayed in her pyjamas some of the time, and stopped having baths. She had bouts of repetitious statements which would become very loud and intrusive and on a few occasions the living room furniture was damaged during aggressive outbursts. All of this was uncharacteristic of Ginger's early development and adulthood.

The psychiatrist was frustrated because Ginger wouldn't talk when she was there, and in his frustration, Mum said, he'd complained that Mum and Dad were doing too much for her. According to Mum's understanding, the psychiatrist felt that Ginger needed to be 'made' to get out and do things, and that her mother needed to stop talking on Ginger's behalf. He reportedly felt Ginger was 'attention-seeking' and that the family were giving in to her too easily. He became irritated, the family felt, with their visits to him, and within a few months he said there was no more he could do for them. At this stage, Ginger was not on any medication and appeared to be very sad indeed. She seemed to be becoming more and more quiet, not making an effort to eat or talk.

The first time I met Ginger and her outgoing, energetic parents in their home, Ginger was dressed, even with make-up, and ready to talk to me, which impressed me very much. I remember spending a lot of time just talking to her about the details of how she not only got herself out of bed, but managed to get dressed and make the extra effort to put make-up on. That line of questioning gave me an idea of quite a few resources that were already present in Ginger, and we had a starting point for getting to her preferred future.

I noticed during the first appointment that Ginger's mum was pretty neurotypical, in as much as she was very tuned in to emotions and to social cues. Also, Ginger's siblings were outgoing, extroverted types as well, which is lovely in itself, but tends to make a person with AS appear even more disabled than they really are. Ginger's father was more like her, though even he was more neurotypical in his views than Ginger was. When I meet a predominantly neurotypical family with one person who has AS, it is both good news and bad news from my point of view. The good news is that the neurotypical family members usually have a good social support network, are resilient, and are able to fight for their AS family member on a number of levels in order to get the needed support. Because of their social skills, it is easy and very pleasant to interact with them. On the other hand, neurotypical family members do tend to judge the AS person by their own standards. The outgoing nature of everyone else makes the person with AS appear even more odd than they really are sometimes. Sadly, it is easy for neurotypical family members to become very upset by things the AS person says because it is easy for them to read emotion into what are intended to be factual statements. In such families, the neurotypical person has to think about everything they say, and about everything they hear from the AS person, and vice versa, because their natural interpretations and expectations will most likely not be right.

This was somewhat the case with Ginger and her family. Mum, who was the main carer, became very quickly upset when Ginger wouldn't get dressed in the morning. She did feel she needed to justify her daughter's behaviour or to pass comment on it quite a lot of the time, which may have made things a bit worse for Ginger than they needed to be. She said, for example, 'Don't say that!' when Ginger said she wished she was dead, which is an understandable temptation for anyone really. Ginger, however, responded better when I said, 'I understand that right now you feel so bad that you wish you weren't here anymore,' because telling her not to say something was perceived as getting at her, and only made her more angry. Part of my preferred future for the family was hearing Mum say things that showed she accepted Ginger's behaviours for just what they were, rather than adding emotion and becoming upset herself. I felt that when Mum started to use different words to talk to Ginger in times of stress, we would be moving in the right direction. I checked this goal with Ginger at about my third visit with her, and she wryly agreed that sometimes Mum became 'very big with emotion'.

Ginger wouldn't go out to appointments so social services came to the house, but then Ginger wouldn't agree to another appointment, so they never came back; Mum wanted them to come unannounced because Ginger would talk to them if she didn't know they were coming. They wouldn't do that, though, as it was apparently against her right to decide about appointments or something. Mum knew that if a support worker said 'We're going here today' Ginger would go, but if asked 'Do you want to…?' Ginger would say no. One of the things I was careful to do, in my solution focused way, was to listen to what Mum said would work, then do that in the belief that she knew Ginger and what Ginger would respond to better than I ever would. Turns out, Mum was right nearly all the time.

At Mum's suggestion, I adopted the idea of telling Ginger I would be in the neighbourhood next Friday, and might call around if I had time, just for a cup of tea and to see if things had improved any. This seemed to work, and I started calling round when I was 'on my way to some stables' (Ginger was a horse fanatic like my good self) and I wondered if Ginger would accompany me so I didn't have to go alone. On these trips, away from Mum and Dad, Ginger certainly did talk. The psychiatrist would have been pleased with her if he'd had this opportunity. Ginger was a great observer and knew how upset Mum and Dad were with her behaviour. In fact, she herself was pretty upset with it, but she did not see how any changes could be made.

So here I was, aiming for my eighth visit with Ginger, who had recently started another medication. I arrived a little early, which startled even the cat, who was waiting on the step to get in. Standing on the step exchanging pleasantries with the cat, I heard a bit of Ginger shouting at her mum and dad before I knocked on the door. It sounded like Ginger was refusing to see me and was threatening to go back to bed. As soon as I knocked on the door, everything went quiet within and the cat and I exchanged glances, awaiting the next event. Mum answered the door, with Ginger smiling behind her. How quickly things changed! We went into the living room, and while Mum was making a drink for me, I asked Ginger how she managed to finish being angry and put on such a polite smile so very quickly! I was truly impressed with not only her ability to do this, but her motivation to do it too. It suggested, and she confirmed that this was so, that she was concerned about what I thought of her.

On this particular day Ginger would not go out with me, so we spent a half an hour talking about things that had been better over the past week. It was a difficult conversation because Ginger said things were better if she stayed in bed all day, but her mother didn't like her doing this. Ginger would get out of bed to go to town with Mum, but only to one shop, where she would want to buy several of the same CDs that she already had at home, and which she would never listen to. This ended in aggravation from Mum too.

In her present state of sadness and anxiety, Ginger was in no position to try understanding things from her mother's point of view. Therefore the best course of action seemed to be to settle things down and take some of the high emotion out of situations. This was a tall order for the family because, I guess, they could see no improvement in sight and were worried that Ginger might be 'stuck' like this for the rest of her life. It is hard to do the little things during a day with a big worry like this weighing you down. All we needed, from my solution focused perspective, was one little change that would unstick things and allow bigger changes to occur. Alas, that one little change did not arrive during this visit.

Ginger's anxiety and tearfulness continued, and about the best success I could claim was that I had been flexible enough to be around when the family was in crisis, I could calm the crisis behaviour a little, Ginger and I had quite a few good visits to animals, and mostly pleasant time which she would not have had otherwise. Also, solution focused thinking enabled me to establish a working relationship with her and her family that had eluded other professionals.

Sadly, however, Ginger stopped seeing me before any significant improvements were made in her mood. She did stop the aggression towards her family and toward property, which was great, but she continued to be sad. Her family decided that they would give her a break from seeing me (it was expensive) until her mood lifted.

Tuesday Evening Social Club

On two Tuesdays of each month I get to meet, at a community centre reserved just for us, with other people of like minds. This started about four years ago. The kind and benevolent mother of one of my ex-clients asked me if I knew any adults who would like to meet on a Saturday and do arts or crafts. As it happened, I knew several somebody's who would like to do anything other than sit alone in their flat or at home with Mum and Dad. Through my practice, I was meeting very many people who were so clever, fun, thoughtful and interesting that it seemed a shame for them not to meet each other. As these things go, one thing led to another thing and the Tuesday Evening Social Club (TESC) was formed. We started meeting once a month but had to double the number of meeting times after about a year because so many people were interested to come, and because we were finding so many interesting things to do.

We have about fifty members, all of whom would describe themselves as somewhat outside 'normal' for one reason or another. There are three people who know where the keys, alarms and equipment are kept, and one of these three opens the centre for us. We have a chairperson, vice-chairperson and secretary, plus 'shadow' appointments of each of these positions. We have a bank account because people keep giving us money and because we started charging fifty pence per person per night to cover refreshment costs.

TESC has a life of its own, and I would be hard-pressed to name any one person who actually runs the thing. I am a common factor because I know everyone who is invited to join so that I can ensure that any vulnerable adults are not vulnerable when they are with us. In that sense the group is not open, and we do not advertise our location or meeting times publicly. Sometimes people think I 'run' the group, but I can assure you that is not the case. A lot of the time, I colour pictures and talk to people. The group runs itself really. It is very much like a birthday party for grown-up kids because everyone can do whatever they want and no one minds. People can sit in a corner observing, can work on computers, can bake, can do crafty things, can kick a ball around, listen to music or just talk. AS is not a requirement, which I particularly like, because people with learning disabilities or mental illness can be just as much fun as people with autism. Parents come sometimes too, but it would be a grave mistake to think the group is run by them! They are there to escape from their role as carers. Some of the parents colour a mean picture, I can tell you.

What I hoped would happen actually did happen, and I would like to see even more of it. That is that TESC members make friends and do things in smaller groups outside of our regular meetings. People visit each other's houses, go to the cinema, go shopping, and talk to each other on the phone. One of the things about TESC that has amazed me, and there are many, is just how social people with AS actually are. For some people, a structure needs to be in place for them to know who to talk to and when to say something. TESC provides a great way for us to practise things like turn-taking and appropriate topics of conversation. We also talk about how to know if someone is a friend, how to meet a stranger, and other kinds of things, and the group has asked me if I can do something in these social skill areas more formally in the future.

We also organize trips out shopping, bowling, barbequeing and looking around museums...you know the sort of thing. One of the things that tickles me when I go along on these trips, which I do not always do, is how the group looks after each other. We seem to ebb and flow around each other so that the people who need support in finding a loo or paying for something, for example, have just what they need when they need it. This is mainly done, it seems by some collective intelligence the group has, because we do not discuss who is going to do what in the way one might for a school outing.

An example of this happened in the Museum of Science and Industry a few weeks ago, when one of the men from our group went to the loo. Apparently this man finds it difficult to stop washing his hands once he starts, consequently he spends a long time in the loo. I was gawping at some display when two members of our group, Eileen and Tom (who have AS and learning disabilities and would not naturally be credited with a 'caretaking' role) looked at their watches and noted that Gareth had been in the loo a long time. Eileen suggested to Tom that he go in and have a look what Gareth was up to, which Tom went and did. Tom came back and said to Eileen that he had given Gareth two minutes to finish washing his hands and come out. (Hell's bells, I thought to myself, how did you know how to do that, Tom?). While we were waiting another man from our group, Marcus, joined us and he offered to go with Tom to get Gareth. I watched with interest because I knew Gareth's 'diagnosis' and I knew it might be difficult for him to be escorted out of the loo. In a short time, the three of them emerged, talking about where they were going to go next in the museum. Such skill. Such sensitivity. Such bloody common sense! And, sadly, the skills Tom, Eileen, Gareth and Marcus used to such good effect in a real-life situation will rarely be noticed by their professionals or their support staff, because we do not think to ask enough about things our clients do well.

Epilogue

This ends our time together, dear reader. We hope you have taken at least one thing from this book that will allow you to do something different and make a positive change in your life. We are interested to hear from readers who wish to contact us, and leave our contact details below:

Missing Link Support Service, Ltd
Support for People Disabled by Society
E. Veronica (Vicky) Bliss
Managing Director/Psychologist

Clarks Cottage
Union Lane
Pilling, Lancs PR3 6SS
0797 156 9042

feedback@missinglinksupportservice.co.uk
ww.missinglinksupportservice.co.uk

Remember: 'Ask the next question. Keep on asking questions and don't stop, and sooner or later you'll be asking intelligent ones. If you live long enough.' (Spider Robinson 1994, p.110)

References

Department of Health (2006) 'Better services for people with an autistic spectrum disorder: A note clarifying current Government policy and describing good practice.' Available at www.dh.gov.uk/Publicationsandstatistics (accessed 6 August 2007)

Robinson, Spider (1994) *Off the Wall at Callahans*. New York: Tor Publishers.

Chapter Seven

Practical Resources

This final section of the book contains resources that might help you if you want to try some solution focused work with someone.

Session Summary Sheet

This is intended for the briefest of note-taking. There are spaces with cues for the worker to help facilitate a solution focused conversation. The first set of boxes is intended for overall, general summary words, followed by the table for smaller, immediately achievable objectives. These would include the sorts of answers a worker might get to questions like 'What will you notice when you take one small step towards where you want to be?' or 'What will one step up on the scale look like?' True to solution focused work, there are three possible scaling scenarios which may be useful. It is often helpful for the therapist to take a few minutes to compose their summary statements and compliments, which can be recorded on the third page. After the session, if the worker has noted any particular successes or difficulties with the therapy session, they can make note of these under the 'Comments on Process of Session' section.

We have included a completed sample of this form.

The Session Summary Sheet is reproduced with kind permission of Brief Solution Pty Ltd., Kurrajong, NSW, Australia.

Session Summary Sheet

Person's name: Jimminey cricket Date: 12-07-07

Current situation (e.g. reason for referral; things to change…)	Preferred Future at End of Therapy
• No energy • crying every day • Do not like where I live	• Go full week without crying • Have a plan to move
Current resources, strengths, coping skills…)	**Who will notice positive changes?**
• Very funny • Have few thousand pounds saved • Have family help • Have methodical approach to problems • Has hope that he can feel better	• J will! • My mum will • Maybe other people J doesn't know yet

Small Changes	Specific examples, steps, what will be happening, etc.
J will get through one evening without crying	J will watch TV in the evening until bed time
J will try to find good things to do	J will read at least a chapter of a novel in an evening
J will visit my mum two times in the week	J might tell her about the book I am reading or J might even make her a meal
	J might try to go out for a walk or cook something new

Exceptions (times when parts of the miracle have already happened, or when the problem isn't so bad...) crys when bored or at lose ends; Has in the past filled time enjoyably by cooking, reading, being on computer, watching DVD's; does not cry when with mother; finds evenings worst time

Overall Feeling Today	What is 'good enough'	Level of Confidence that your goals can be achieved
10	10	10
9	9	9
8	8 ✔	8
7	7	7
6	6	6 ✔
5	5	5
4 ✔	4	4
3	3	3
2	2	2
1	1	1
0	0	0

Scaling (10 = best ever/0 = worst ever)

End of session message

Summary and compliments	Task
Even though feeling tired and blue, J came for appointment AND made the effort to answer all my questions! Despite feeling low, J remains hopeful that he can make some positive changes J has solved many problems and survived low periods before, so has a lot of experience in this area	None suggested by me. J has given himself some tasks as noted above. Made suggestion that J might look out for mum's reaction if she notices that he's a bit happier.

Comments on process of session

J turned up on time and worked hard to make the most of the time we had.

Had feeling that J was working as hard as I was to find a way forward.

J seemed relaxed with the approach, and seemed to appreciate taking time to identify his existing strengths.

conversation was especially easy when we were talking about the times when he is NOT crying or tired or sad.

Next appointment: J decided to book a return appointment in 3 weeks' time

Therapist: ____________________

Session Summary Sheet

Person's name: ________________ Date: ________________

Current situation (e.g. reason for referral; things to change…)	Preferred Future at End of Therapy
Current resources, strengths, coping skills…)	Who will notice positive changes?

Small Changes	**Specific examples, steps, what will be happening, etc.**

Exceptions (times when parts of the miracle have already happened, or when the problem isn't so bad…)

Overall Feeling Today	What is 'good enough'	Level of Confidence that your goals can be achieved
10	10	10
9	9	9
8	8	8
7	7	7
6	6	6
5	5	5
4	4	4
3	3	3
2	2	2
1	1	1
0	0	0

Scaling (10 = best ever/0 = worst ever)

End of session message

Summary and compliments	Task

Comments on process of session

Next appointment: ____________________

Therapist: ____________________

Scaling Record

This one page graph is intended to keep track of a person's ratings over time. The scales can, of course, be adapted to suit the needs of each individual, but in the example given we used an overall rating of how the person was feeling in themselves. One could equally keep a record of the level of hope a person has that they will improve, or the level of confidence they have that the therapist can help them, or any of a number of things.

We have completed one summary as an example.

Summary of How I Am Doing

Name: Jimminey cricket

Date	04-07-07	31-07-07	19-08-07	12-09-07	31-10-07
10 = Things are the absolute best they can be ☺☺☺					
9					
8					✔
7				✔	
6					
5 = Things are OK ☺		✔			
4	✔		✔		
3					
2					
1					
0 = Things are the very worst they could be ☹☹☹					

Summary of How I Am Doing

Name: ____________________

Date					
10 = Things are the absolute best they can be ☺☺☺					
9					
8					
7					
6					
5 = Things are OK ☺					
4					
3					
2					
1					
0 = Things are the very worst they could be ☹☹☹					

Rating Sheets

The next two forms are simple rating scales of four items each. The first, an Overall Rating Form, can be used to help the worker and client decide what areas of the person's life are going well, and what areas might be good to talk about during the session. In the example we have given, the person was referred because of a decrease in productivity at work. The person's supervisor felt that the person was becoming less attentive to his job and was therefore making too many errors. Upon completing the Overall Rating Form, however, it becomes clear that the person themselves felt work was going well, but that family life was not as good as he would like.

Some people will struggle to use this type of form, so the worker needs to check out the ratings by wording the options in different ways, and by checking whether or not the overall rating appears to make sense given the individual ratings on the other three items. Workers can modify the scales by using fewer numbers or by using perhaps a big box to signify happy and a small box to signify less happy.

The second rating scale, 'About our Work Today', provides a nice summary of a client's view of the session they have just had. It could be used for a therapy session, but equally for a cooking lesson or even a day out with a few changes in the wording. People with autism are usually pretty forthright in giving their opinions, so the worker needs to be of a strong constitution to ask for these ratings!

How Are You – Rating Sheet

Name: Jimminey cricket Age (Yrs) 45

Session Number 1 Session Date 01-07-07

Looking back *over the last week, including today,* rate how well you have been doing in the following areas of your life, where marks to the top indicate pretty happy and marks towards the bottom mean less happy. We might use this to decide what to talk about today.

You in yourself	You with your family	You with your friends or people at work or school	Overall
☺ Best ever	☺ Best ever	☺ Best ever	☺ Best ever
5	5	5 (circled)	5
4	4	4	4
3	3	3	3 (circled)
2 (circled)	2	2	2
1	1 (circled)	1	1
Worst ever ☹	Worst ever ☹	Worst ever ☹	Worst ever ☹

How Did We Do – Rating Sheet

Name: Jimminey cricket Age (Yrs) 45

Session Number 1 Session Date 01-07-07

The therapist aims to listen to you, work on things of importance to you and help you plan a way forward in a way that is right for you. Circle a number which shows how well you think the therapist did.

I felt heard, understood and respected	We worked on and talked about what I wanted to work on and talk about	I am taking something useful from today's session	Overall, today's meeting was right for me
☺ Very much	☺ Absolutely	☺ Absolutely	☺ Absolutely
5 (circled)	5	5	5
4	4 (circled)	4 (circled)	4 (circled)
3	3	3	3
2	2	2	2
1	1	1	1
Not at all ☹	Not at all ☹	Not at all ☹	Not at all ☹

How Are You – Rating Sheet

Name: ____________________ Age (Yrs) _____

Session Number __________ Session Date _____________

Looking back *over the last week, including today,* rate how well you have been doing in the following areas of your life, where marks to the top indicate pretty happy and marks towards the bottom mean less happy. We might use this to decide what to talk about today.

You in yourself	**You with your family**	**You with your friends or people at work or school**	**Overall**
☺ Best ever	☺ Best ever	☺ Best ever	☺ Best ever
5	5	5	5
4	4	4	4
3	3	3	3
2	2	2	2
1	1	1	1
Worst ever ☹	Worst ever ☹	Worst ever ☹	Worst ever ☹

How Did We Do – Rating Sheet

Name: ____________________ Age (Yrs) _____

Session Number _________ Session Date _____________

The therapist aims to listen to you, work on things of importance to you and help you plan a way forward in a way that is right for you. Circle a number which shows how well you think the therapist did.

I felt heard, understood and respected	**We worked on and talked about what I wanted to work on and talk about**	**I am taking something useful from today's session**	**Overall, today's meeting was right for me**
☺ Very much	☺ Absolutely	☺ Absolutely	☺ Absolutely
5	5	5	5
4	4	4	4
3	3	3	3
2	2	2	2
1	1	1	1
Not at all ☹	Not at all ☹	Not at all ☹	Not at all ☹

Solution Focused Note Sheet

This worksheet gives the solution focused worker a fairly comprehensive 'cheat' sheet of questions to ask along with space to make note of memorable aspects of the interview. We think the form is self-explanatory and would like to thank BRIEF (7–8 Newbury Street, London EC1A 7HU, Tel: 020 7600 3366, www.brieftherapy.org.uk) along with Harry Korman for giving us the background on which this resource is based.

A Solution Focused Note Sheet

Remember:

1. Ask questions that people have a chance of answering.
2. Ask questions to which you do not already know the answers.
3. *Always* check your understanding of what the client says.
4. Clients must recognise their resources – not the therapist.
5. Initially we want to agree a 'common project'
    - something client wants done
    - which is within my remit
    - which we can actually do if we work together.
6. It is helpful for people to know *what will be different* when their problem is managed so that they know when things are improving.
7. People who describe the way they want things to be *in great detail* are more likely to get it.

1. **Presenting problem** (client's own words, referrer's problem, etc.):

2. Problem-free talk:

- I know very little about you apart from what brings you here today. What would you feel happy to tell me about yourself?
- What are you interested in?
- What do you enjoy?
- What are you good at?
- What about your family?
- How would your best friend describe you?

3. Pre-treatment change:

- Often between making an appointment and arriving for that appointment people have already noticed a change. Have you noticed any changes?

4. **Best hopes for the session:**
   - How will you know that it was useful coming here today?
   - What will it take for you to say that this has been worthwhile?

5. **Preferred future:**
   - Imagine that after you have gone to bed tonight a miracle happens and the problems that brought you here today are resolved. But since you are asleep you will not know that the miracle has happened. When you wane up tomorrow morning, what will be different that will tell you a miracle has happened?
   - What will you see yourself doing differently?
   - What will others see you doing?
   - How will your mum/dad/teacher know that the miracle has happened?
   - What will be the first sign of the miracle happening?
   - What small step would be a sign of moving in the right direction or being on the right track?
   - How will you know that life is going well for you?
   - What will tell you that you don't need to come here any more?
   - Imagine a day going well, how will you know the day is going well?
   - And if this problems were resolved, what would be differnet in your life that would tell you?

- Just imagine that this probation order turns out to be more useful that you thought it would, how will you know? What will be different in your life?
- How will you know that this placement has been useful to you (or your child)?
- Imagine that you take back control of your life from (depression, anger, alcohol) how will you know that you are living a life that does you justice?

6. Exceptions:

- When are the times when this isn't a problem?
- When are the times that it doesn't last as long?
- When are the times that it seems to be less intense?
- When are the times that you feel better?
- When are the times that it bothers you least?
- When do you resist the urge to…?

7. Coping:

- So what has been helping you to survive?
- How have you been getting through?
- How come you have not given up hope?
- So how have you managed to get here today?
- What do you think your best friend, for example, most admires about the way that you have been struggling with this?
- How do you cope?
- That situation sounds pretty overwhelming; how do you get by?
- What do you do that helps you to get through?
- What is it that gives you the strength to even get up in the morning?

8. Stopping Things Getting Worse:

- So what have you been doing to stop things getting even worse?
- So how come you aren't at (e.g.) minus three on your scale?
- You say that things have gone down on the scale. What did you do to stop the slide at (e.g.) four?

9. Scales:

- On a scale of zero to ten, with zero being the worst that things have been in your life, and ten being how you want things to be, where are you today?
- So what is it that you are doing that means that you are at … and not at zero?
- So if you are on three tell me what you will be doing that will tell you when you are four?
- Who will be the first person to notice when you have moved up a point on the scale?
- Where on that scale represents 'good enough' for you? The point that you would settle for? How will you know you are at that point on the scale?
- On a scale of zero to ten where would you rate your desire for change?
- What would be happening when it is one point higher?
- How would you rate your confidence that you can make a change?
- How confident do you feel that you can keep others and yourself safe?
- If you were to move up one point on your behaviour scale, what difference might this make to your relationship with your mum?

10. Locating resources, building on strengths:

- When you faced this sort of problem in the past, how did you resolve it?
- How would you know that you were doing that again?
- What other tough situations have you handled?
- What did handling that well tell you about yourself?
- What is your approach to finding solutions to tough situations?
- If you read about a woman who had been through what you have been through what do you imagine you would think of her?

11. View of self:

- What does this achievement teach you about yourself?
- What do you now know about yourself that you didn't know last week?
- Whas that a surprise to you?
- What have you learned from this experience?
- What have you learned from this experience that will be useful to you in your future?

12. Constructive history:

- Who would be least surprised by this change that you have made, this achievement?
- What did that person know about you that others did not know?
- How do the qualities that you drew on to make this change relate to the qualities of other members of your family?
- What in the past have you achieved that is in some way similar to this?
- Looking back what tells you that you always were capable of doing this?
- When else, in the past, have you noticed yourself drawing on similar qualities?
- Have you always been a survivor or did you have to learn the hard way?
- It sounds like you needed to look after yourself from a very early age – when did you first realize you had the capacity to do this?
- I can see it has been very hard to show love to your children, but when did you first realize that even though it was hidden, that love was there?
- How do you manage to keep your sense of humour – is this one of the qualities you have which has kept you doing?

Solution Focused Workbook

This workbook was put together by Vicky for use with some clients who particularly like art/craft work. It is very basic in order to allow for the creativity of both the worker and the client to make the book applicable to themselves and their work together. In a few instances it has been helpful for Vicky to complete one workbook with her view of the client while the client completes their own with their view of themselves, and then to compare the two books. People with autism often do not know what other people think of them, and this workbook provides a structure for the worker to show how many positive things they have noticed and appreciated about the client.

Photographs, magazine pictures, beads, craft papers, stickers and all manner of creative things can be used to make completion of the book interesting. Some people prefer to complete the book on their own and others prefer to complete it during sessions with a worker. Often people are more apt to talk about themselves while engaged in an activity, and this book can provide a useful structured activity over which interesting conversations can be held.

Solution Focused Workbook

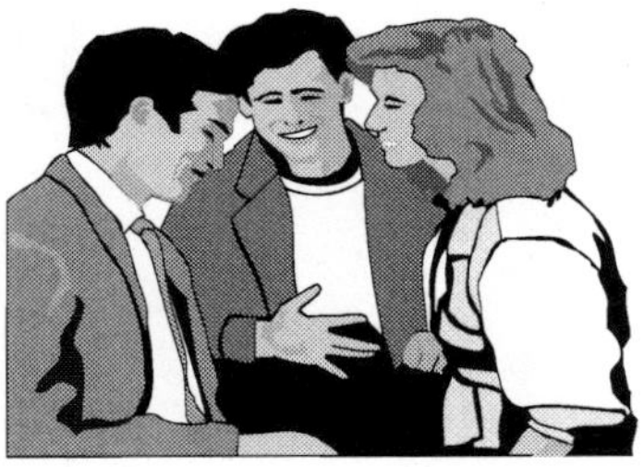

This book belongs to:

____

With help from

____

____

____

Date(s)

____

____

What is this book about?

You have asked for help because there are things in your life that you would like to change.

Part of the book will help us to learn more about *you* and how things are for you now.

Part of the book will help us to learn what it is that would make you feel better.

Part of the book will help us to learn the things you are already doing that are working for you.

What will we do?

We will talk, write or draw about things in as much detail as possible.

It might seem that we ask a lot of hard questions!

Remember: People who are able to say what they want will most often get it!

What are some problems you have faced?

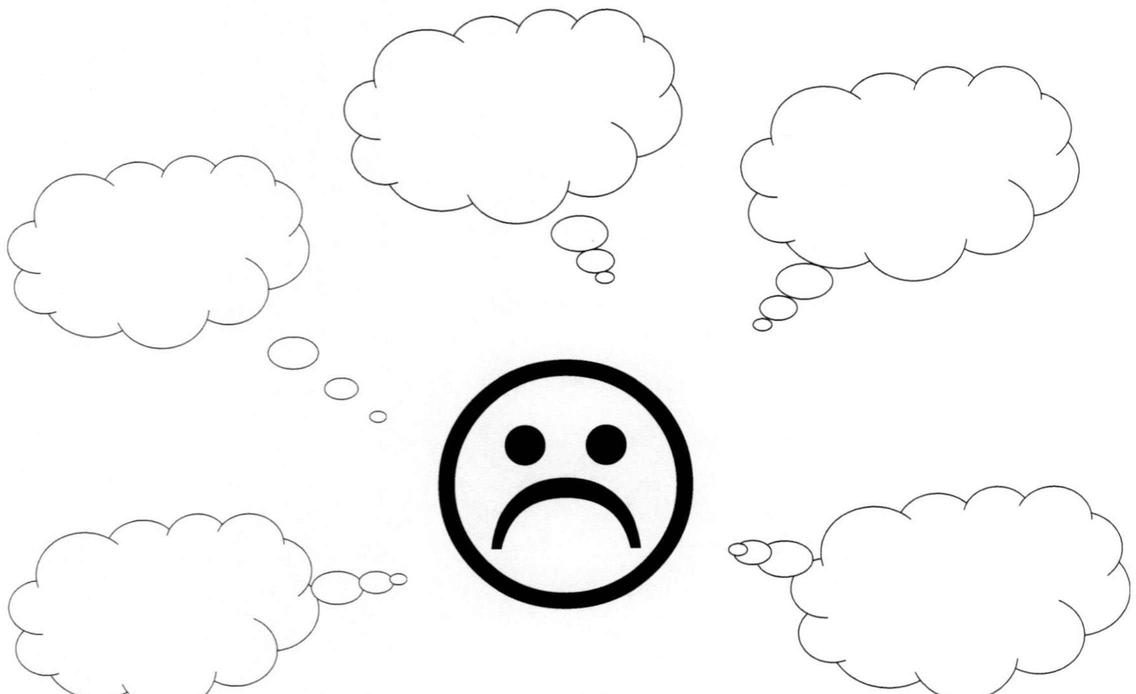

What are the main things bothering you at this time?

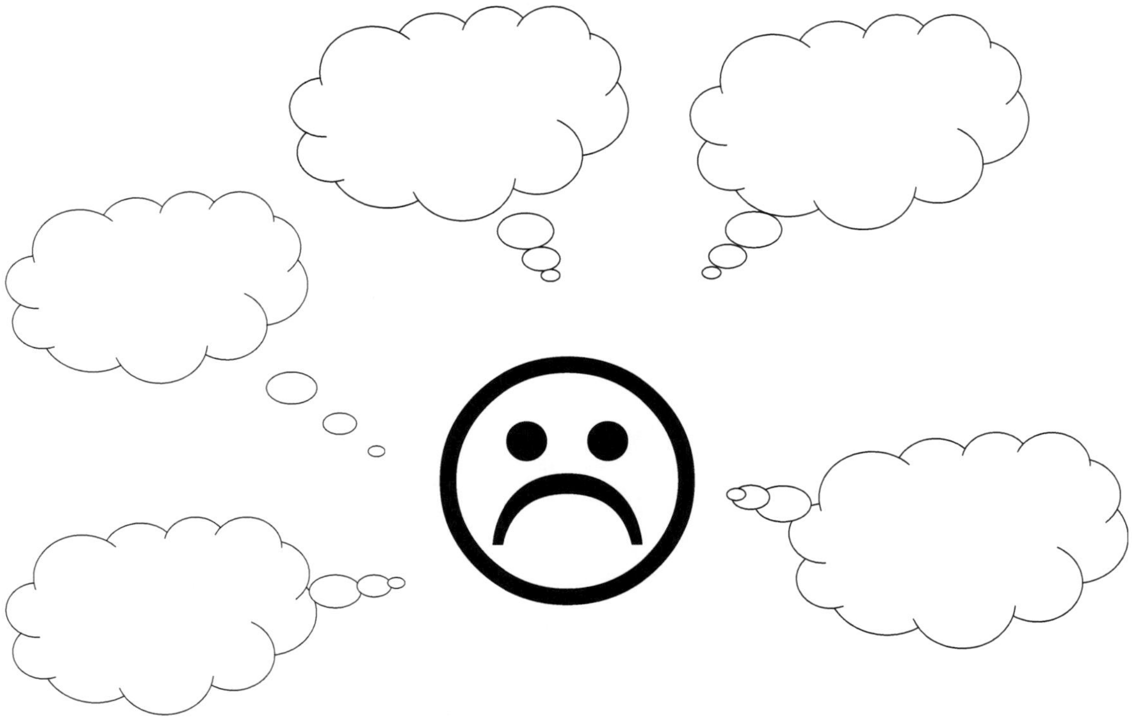

What are your *best* hopes for our work together?

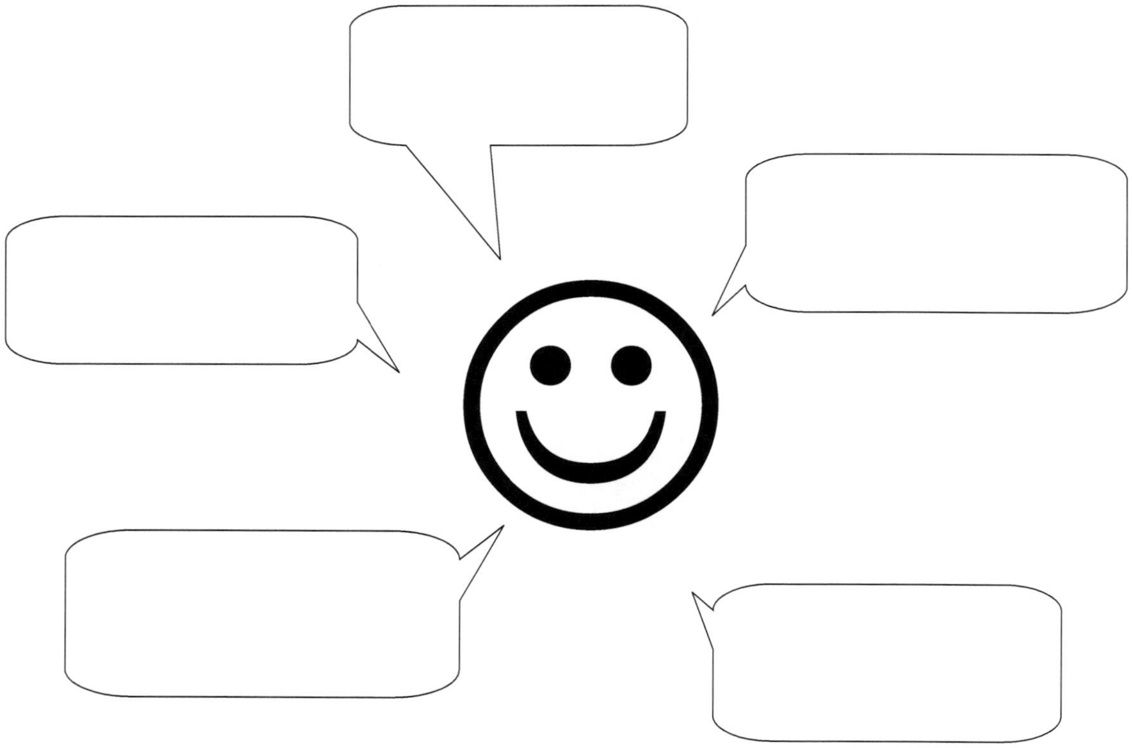

Write some important things about yourself

Write about your history and some of the things you have achieved in your life.

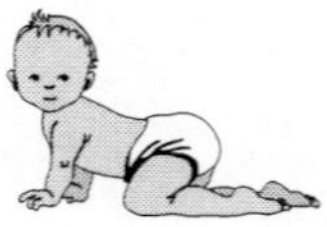

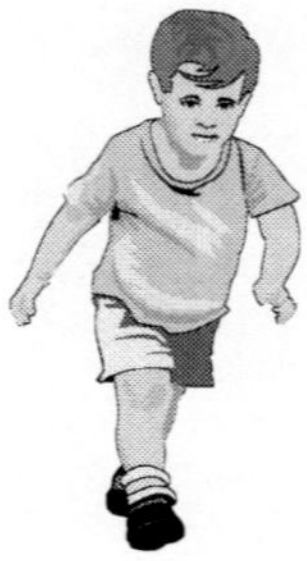

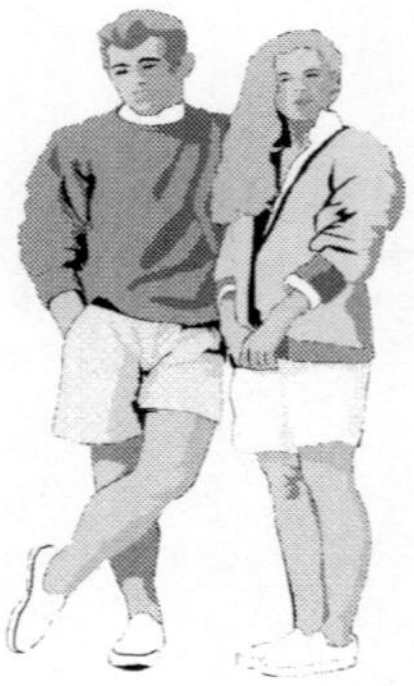

Pretend a miracle happens whilst you are asleep tonight.

What will be different for you tomorrow when you wake up?

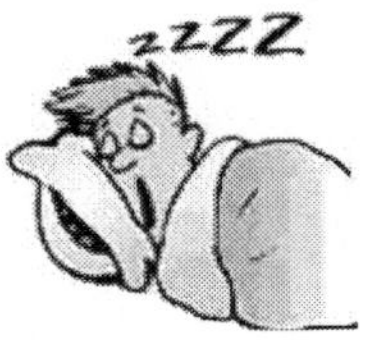

When are the times when the problems aren't there or are less troublesome?

What has helped you to manage the problems?

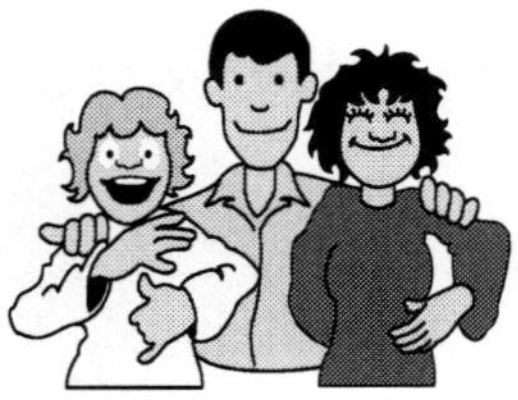

How have you stopped things getting even worse?

When you've faced problems before, how did you cope with them?

What does coping with all these problems tell you about yourself?

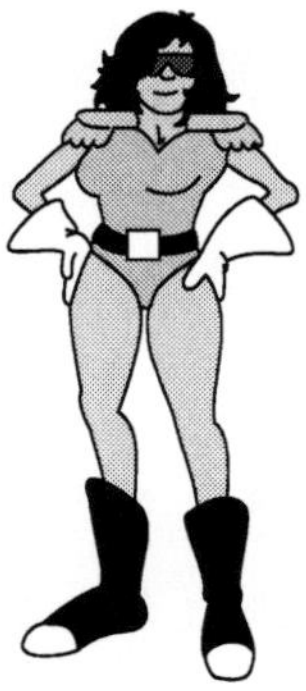

Write some of the good things that have happened since we last met

Good things ☺	What this tells me about myself ☹

Index

20020025R00090

Printed in Great Britain
by Amazon